Viscoelastics in Ophthalmic Surgery

Springer

Berlin
Heidelberg
New York
Barcelona
Hong Kong
London
Milano
Paris
Singapore
Tokyo

H. B. Dick · O. Schwenn

Viscoelastics
in Ophthalmic Surgery

With 147 Figures, some in Color

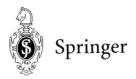
Springer

Priv.-Doz. Dr. med. H. Burkhard Dick
Department of Ophthalmology
Johannes Gutenberg-University
Langenbeckstrasse 1, D-55131 Mainz
Germany

Dr. med. Oliver Schwenn
Department of Ophthalmology
Johannes Gutenberg-University
Langenbeckstrasse 1, D-55131 Mainz
Germany

ISBN 3-540-67330-X Springer-Verlag Berlin Heidelberg New York

Library of Congress Cataloging-in-Publication Data

Dick, H. Burkhard: Viscoelastics in ophthalmic surgery / H.B. Dick ; O. Schwenn. – Berlin; Heidelberg;
New York; Barcelona; Hong Kong; Milano; Paris; Singapore; Tokyo : Springer, 2000
    ISBN 3-540-67330-X

Springer-Verlag is a company in the BertelsmannSpringer publishing group
© Springer-Verlag Berlin Heidelberg 2000
Printed in Germany

Cover design: *design & production* GmbH, Heidelberg
Typesetting: Goldener Schnitt, Sinzheim
Printed on acid-free paper – SPIN: 10723820   18/3134   5 4 3 2 1 0

Foreword

It will be difficult to find an ophthalmic surgeon who will gladly do his work entirely without viscoelastics. Within just a few years this group of substances has enlarged the field of ophthalmic surgery enormously. Many procedures have become safer and simpler and other techniques could only be developed because of the availability of viscoelastics. Especially cataract surgery and implantation of intraocular lenses have benefitted. Implantation of an intraocular lens can be performed much more reliably into the capsular bag without endangering the posterior capsule. Implantation of foldable lenses would be almost impossible without viscoelastics. However, other surgical maneuvers also necessitate viscoelastics, especially when the anterior chamber must be maintained, the corneal endothelium must be protected and delicate tissues must be manipulated. A corneal transplant can be sutured safely into the recipient corneal ring using viscoelastics. Even in glaucoma surgery, viscoelastics gain importance as they are being used in trabeculectomy or in deep sclerectomy with additional viscocanalostomy.

But which substance is best for which purpose? Just as much as a basic pharmacological knowledge is necessary for a rational use of drugs, in-depth knowledge of physicochemical properties and objective investigations are prerequisites for a logical selection of viscoelastics from an ever increasing number of available substances.

H. Burkhard Dick and Oliver Schwenn, both ophthalmologists at the department of ophthalmology at Mainz university, have embarked on the enterprise to systematically investigate viscoelastics and to collect the necessary knowledge. They present the basic principals and properties of substances and an up to date selection of the techniques that can be performed using viscoelastics. This book is going to be a standard text and the reference for any viscoelastic which is available at present or will be available in the future. The book contains a precise presentation of the basics as well as a survey of practical and clinical information. Without any doubt it will find many thankful readers.

Prof. Dr. med. Norbert Pfeiffer
Chairman
Department of Ophthalmology
University of Mainz, Germany

Acknowledgements

Our special appreciation goes to Prof. Dr. Tadeusz Pakula as well as to Mr. Thomas Hirschmann in the Max-Planck-Institute for Polymeric Research (Mainz) at the Department of Rheology for their constructive hints, everlasting willingness for discussions, and active support when investigating and calculating the properties of viscoelastic substances.

A very special thanks is extended to our academic teacher and medical director of the eye clinic of the University Mainz Prof. Dr. med. Norbert Pfeiffer.

Our gratitude goes to Mrs. Marlene Maser-Wahle and Mrs. Martina Pfeiffer for their supportive engagement with some illustrations. We extend our appreciation and thanks to Mrs. Dr. S. Petrou-Binder (Frankfurt/M.), Dr. M.U. Drüsedau (Plau am See) for the helpful revision of our manuscript. We are indepted to the head-photographer Axel Welsch for the pleasing pictures and photographical art work.

We extend our thanks to all the companies that supplied us with sufficient material of their viscoelastic products for our research (mostly without charging us).

We thank the following companies for supplying us with illustrations: Pharmacia & Upjohn; Alcon Pharma.

Our appreciation is extended to the publishing company Springer-Verlag, we are especially indepted to Mrs. Yvonne Bertram and Mr. Rainer Kusche for their outstanding cooperation and fast completion of this project.

I extend my sincerest appreciation to my teachers for ophtalmic surgery Prof. Dr. med. Dr. h.c. Franz Grehn (medical director of the eye clinic of the University Würzburg) and Dr. med. Bernd Weber (head physician of the eye clinic of the "Bürgerhospital" Frankfurt); sincerely Dr. med. O. Schwenn.

A very special thanks to my partner in life Dr. jur. Astrid Meckel (judge at the Landgericht) for her supportive input for the chapter "Medical device or drug" and her patience and consideration during the preparation of this textbook, thankfully Priv.-Doz. Dr. med. H.B. Dick.

Finally I thank my teacher for ophtalmic surgery and head physician Dr. med. Oliver Schwenn.

H. Burkhard Dick
Oliver Schwenn

Preface

Nowadays viscoelastics are applied in almost every cataract operation and in many other ophthalmic surgeries. It is hard to think of related fields and surgical steps whithout viscoelastic substances. Everyday we are confronted with a increasing number of new viscoelastic products and accordingly with new surgical techniques. Last but not least recent research results present a number of new facts which are not always easy to correlate to the actions in the clinical field. Qualified handling of viscoelastics however is impossible without the foundation of knowledge and without relation to practical matters clinical research will not be successful. The main purpose of this book was to give a critical overview about all aspects of the possible application of viscoelastics. It imparts updated basic knowledge as well as practical information and experiences concerning clinical matters. We tried to emphasize on combining updated basic knowledge and comparative studies with easy to understand information of practical relevance. Important fresh impetus was added to this project due to the interdisciplinary research cooperation with the Max-Planck-Institute for Polymeric research, department of rheology, in Mainz, Germany. This book adresses beginning as well as experienced ophthalmic surgeons.

Mainz, April 2000

H. Burkhard Dick
Oliver Schwenn

Table of Contents

Dedicated to our patients

CHAPTER 1

Overview

Introduction

The development of microsurgical techniques and the perfection of intraocular lens (IOL) implantation has led to a wide-spread acceptance of cataract operations. The number of cataract operations has been rising steadily, worldwide, since the introduction of IOL implantation. In 1999, 430 000 cataract operations were performed in Germany alone, thus establishing cataract operations as the most frequently performed surgical procedure.

One of the most important conditions for IOL implantation in cataract operations is a deep anterior chamber. This condition is essential for microsurgical manipulation in the spacially limited anterior eye segment and ultimately serves to protect the corneal endothelial cells. This single-cell-layer endothelium may be injured during surgery to varying degrees and is known to be incapable of cell regeneration. After the surgical opening of the eye, the anterior chamber normally flattens and completely collapses after a short period of time. In addition to aqueous outflow, a second event is known to contribute to the collapse of the anterior chamber space: increased ocular perfusion pressure and subsequent vascular bed perfusion, in response to the drop in intraocular pressure to zero after eye incision. Consequently, a massive thickening of the choroid vascular bed ensues which drives the vitreous body and the iris-lens-diaphragm forward, resulting in a flat anterior chamber.

Maintaining a deep anterior chamber can be considered the *conditio sine qua non* for successful anterior segment intraocular surgery. There are diverse pre- and intraoperative precautionary measures available to achieve this: oculopression, addition of adrenalin and hyaluronidase to retrobulbar anesthesia, hyperventilation and blood pressure reduction during anesthesia, closed system operation as made possible by phacoemulsification (lens nucleus disintegration via ultrasound), or by intravenous infusion of hyperosmolar substances (Vörösmarthy, 1967; Kelman, 1967).

A definitive advance was made with the introduction of viscoelastic substances in anterior segment surgery (Balazs, 1983; Balazs, 1984; Balazs, 1986). Viscoelastic substances (ophthalmic viscosurgical devices, OVD), a class of nonactive surgical implants with viscous and/or viscoelastic properties were intended for use during surgery in the anterior segment of the eye.

The effects of viscoelastic substances in maintaining the anterior chamber space and the protection offered the vulnerable corneal endothelium from mechanical and surgical traumas have crucially improved the course and results of intraocular anterior segment procedures; thereby, decisively contributing to successful artificial lens implantation in cataract surgery (Glasser et al., 1986; Glasser et al., 1989; Glasser et al., 1991; Holmberg & Philipson, 1984 a and 1984 b; Kerr Muir et al., 1987; MacRae et al., 1983; Polack, 1986; Soll et al., 1980).

Historical Development

Diverse polymers and viscous substances[1] were used earlier in animal and human eyes for endothelial protection and vitreous replacement; none of which, however, proved useful for application in viscosurgery. In 1934, Meyer and Palmer succeeded in isolating a substance from the vitreous humor, which was, henceforth, to be called hyaluronic acid. Endré Balazs (1960) dedicated a large part of his scientific research efforts to the development of artificial vitreous bodies, recognizing hyaluronic acid as an ideal substance. It was this finding which coincidentally led to the implementation of hyaluronic acid in anterior segment surgery. Balazs succeeded in isolating hyaluronic acid from the umbilical cord and rooster combs and developed a more purified version for use in ophthalmology. The highly sensitive owl monkey eye test (see below) was used to recognize endotoxic inflammatory substances. The application of hyaluronic acid in the vitreous space did not, however, bring about the hoped-for success (Balazs, 1960; Balazs & Hutsch, 1976). Miller (1977) employed sodium hyaluronate in experimental implantations in animals. Balazs first reported on hyaluronic acid within the context of anterior segment surgery on the human eye in France in 1979 and patented it in the US for its use in anterior chamber surgery that same year (Balazs, 1979). This US patent was sold to Pharmacia and Upjohn, who developed the first high-molecular viscoelastic, Healon®, for the market in 1979. Healon® was first used as vitreous replacement and found useful as a lubricant in race horses suffering from joint disease. Hyaluronic acid proved most instrumental in anterior segment surgery. Balazs coined the term 'viscosurgery' for surgeries involving the use of viscoelastic solutions.

Georg Eisner (1980, 1981) explored surgical viscoelastic substance use from the more practical aspects of tissue surface application and space creation. His impressive representations of viscoblockade, -tamponade and viscospatula (Eisner, 1983) are a tribute to his efforts.

---

[1] [examples: glycerinemethylacrylate-gel (Daniele, Refojo, Schepens & Freeman, 1968), polyacrylamide-gels (Müller-Jensen, 1974), polygelin (Oosterhuis, Van Haeringen, Jeltes & Glasius, 1966), polyvinylpyrrolidon (Scuderi, 1954), dextransulfate (Gombos & Berman, 1967), carboxymethylcellulose (Kishimoto, Yamanouchi, Mori & Nakamori, 1964), chondroitin sulfate (Kishimoto, Yamanouchi, Mori & Nakamori, 1964; Mori, 1967; Soll & Harrison, 1981; MacRae, Edelhauser, Hyndiuk, Burd & Schultz, 1983), methylcellulose (Fechner, 1977; MacRae, Edelhauser, Hyndiuk, Burd & Schultz, 1983), sodium alginate (Mori, 1967) and collagen (Dunn, Stenzel, Rubin & Miyata, 1969; Pruett, Calabria & Schepens, 1967; Stenzel, Dunn & Rubin, 1969)]

Current Breakdown of Viscoelastic Substances

Following Healon®´s introduction into the market, ophthalmic viscosurgical devices (OVD) experienced both a rapid spread and modification as manufacturers developed an array of substances with diverse formulations.

At the moment, the variety of new viscoelastic preparations is vast and therefore, varies extensively from place to place (Fig. 1).

Steve Arshinoff pointed out the significance of the physical basis of viscoelastic substances with regard to their distinctive nature. He divided them into two groups (Table 1): the high viscous-cohesive and the low viscous-dispersive viscoelastic substances (Arshinoff, 1998). The high viscous group was further subdivided by Arshinoff into highly viscous (>1000 Pas) and viscous (100 Pas< x <1000 Pas) agents. Allervisc® Plus (formerly Ivisc®) and Healon® GV belong to the highly viscous group, while Ivisc®, Allervisc® Plus, Provisc®, Healon®, Biolon®, Allervisc®, Amvisc® and Amvisc® Plus (following an order of decreasing viscosity as determined by the manufacturer) belong to the viscous group. Arshinoff allotted Viscoat®, Cellugel®, Vitrax®, i-Cell®, Ocuvis®, Ocucoat®, Hymecel®, Adatocel®, and Visilon® to the medium viscous or low viscous-dispersive viscoelastic substances. It should be noted that this simplified breakdown is based on product information provided by the manufacturers and not on independent comparative testing of substance viscosity. Dick, Schwenn and Pfeiffer developed a classification according to independently obtained measurement results in 1999.

Based on our own study results, we propose a partial revision of the viscoelastic substance grouping/classification proposed by Arshinoff, to be based on the rheologic and physicochemical characteristics of viscoelastic substances obtained in cooperation with the Max-Planck Institute for Polymer Research, Department of Rheology, in Mainz, Germany. Furthermore, a new product, the so-called "viscous cohesion dissociated high molecular weight viscoelastic", better known by its product name, Healon®5 (Fig. 2), is now at our disposal. Healon®5 is formulated to fulfill specific requirements for use in phacoemulsification (i.e., with both cohesive and dispersive characteristics).

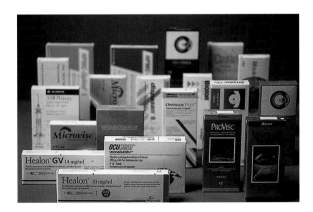

Fig. 1. A selection of commercially available viscoelastic substances in Germany to this date

Table 1. Division of the OVD into two groups (Arshinoff 1995 & 1998)

high viscosity (cohesive)			
viscoelastic substance	content	molecular weight (D)	zero shear viscosity (Pas)
high viscous			
Ivisc® Plus	1.4 % HA	7.9 M	4.8 K
Healon® GV	1.4 % HA	5.0 M	2.0 K
viscous			
Ivisc®	1.0 % HA	6.1 M	1.0 K
Allervisc® Plus	1.4 % HA	5.1 M	500
Provisc®	1.0 % HA	2.0 M	280
Healon®	1.0 % HA	4.0 M	230
Biolon™	1.4 % HA	3.0 M	215
Allervisc®	1.0 % HA	5.1 M	200
Amvisc® Plus	1.2 % HA	1.0 M	100
Amvisc® Plus	1.6 % HA	1.0 M	100
low viscosity (dispersive)			
viscoelastic substance	content	molecular weight (D)	zero shear viscosity (Pas)
medium viscous			
Viscoat®	3.0 % HA	500 K	41
	4.0 % CS	25 K	
Cellugel®	2.0 % HPMC	100 K	38
Vitrax®	3.0 % HA	500 K	25
low viscous			
i-Cell®	2.0 % HPMC	90 K	6
Ocuvis®	2.0 % HPMC	90 K	4.3
Ocucoat®	2.0 % HPMC	86 K	4
Hymecel®	2.0 % HPMC	86 K	4
Adatocel®	2.0 % HPMC	86 K	4
Visiolon®	2.0 % HPMC	86 K	4

M = million, K = thousand, HA = sodium hyaluronate, CS = chondroitin sulfate, $HPMC$ = hydroxypropylmethylcellulose

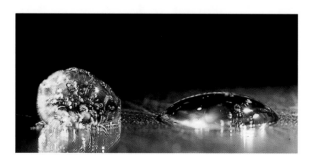

Fig. 2. Comparative picture of Healon®5 (left) and Healon® (right) suggests a difference in physicochemical and rheological properties of these two OVD both containing hyaluronic acid

Analysis of Current Application Modes

A survey made by Leaming (1999) in the US, revealed that over 95% of members of the American Society of Cataract and Refractive Surgery (ASCRS) use hyaluronic acid as the OVD of choice in phacoemulsification (Fig. 3). The majority of OVD surveyed, elected hyaluronic acid as the choice viscoelastic agent in extracapsular cataract extraction as well (Fig. 4), with variations in specific choice of product. Several interesting trends have been observed over the years which dominate the selection of a preferred viscoelastic product (Leaming, 1991-1998). 58% of polled American colleagues use a single viscoelastic substance in phacoemulsification procedures, never using a second; 5% use a second viscoelastic substance routinely; and 37% of ophthalmic surgeons asked, employ a second agent in 1 out of 10 operations (Fig. 5). Approximately 2/3 of American ophthalmic surgeons polled give priority to universally applicable viscoelastics, while 1/5 prefer the use of different viscoelastic substances in different situations (Fig. 6).

Fig. 3. Percentage distribution of preferably used viscoelastic products in phacoemulsification obtained during a survey among 1377 members of the American Society of Cataract and Refractive Surgery (ASCRS, modified according to Leaming, 1999)

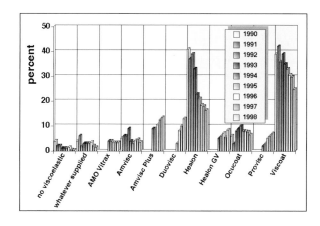

Fig. 4. Percentage distribution of preferably used viscoelastic products in routine extracapsular cataract extractions (ECCE) obtained during a survey among 1328 members of the American Society of Cataract and Refractive Surgery (ASCRS; modified according to Leaming, 1997)

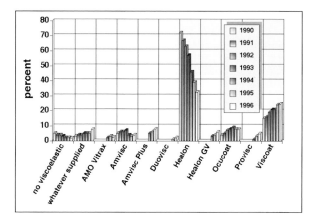

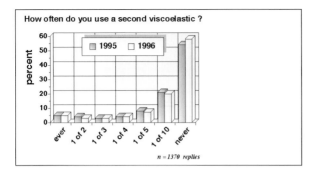

Fig. 5. Percentage distribution of the number of ophthalmic surgeons, who apply a second viscoelastic substance during phacoemulsification obtained during a survey among 1370 members of the American Society of Cataract and Refractive Surgery (ASCRS; modified according to Leaming, 1997)

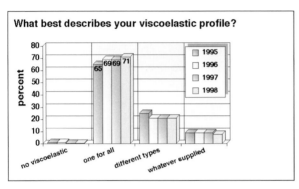

Fig. 6. Percentage distribution of the requested profile of viscoelastic substances that ophthalmic surgeons would prefer. The data was obtained during a survey among 1439 members of the American Society of Cataract and Refractive Surgery (ASCRS; modified according to Leaming, 1999)

In Europe as well, hyaluronic acid is most commonly chosen, followed by hydroxypropylmethylcellulose. In German-speaking countries, a poll taken by Wenzel and co-workers showed a similar preference for hyaluronic acid among the majority of members of the DGII (Deutschsprachige Gesellschaft für Intraokularlinsen-Implantation und Refraktive Chirurgie) (Wenzel, Ohrloff & Duncker, 1998), although 45% of the same group of colleages preferred the use of hydroxypropylmethylcellulose (HPMC) preparations (Figure 7). These poll results show little variation to an earlier inquiry, made by Wenzel and Rochels (1996), in regard to the viscoelastic choice made by ophthalmic surgeons in German-speaking areas. The number of ophthalmic surgeons using gas (air) during IOL implantation has sunk from 5% (1996) to a minimum (1998).

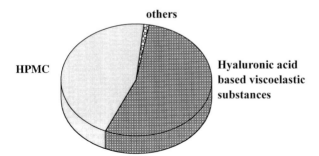

Fig. 7. Percentage distribution of main classes of viscoelastic substances routinely applied during cataract operations. Data for the German speaking areas (modified according to Wenzel et al., 1999)

CHAPTER 2

Basics

Physicochemical Properties of Ophthalmic viscosurgical devices (OVD)

Due to immense product diversity, ophthalmic surgeons rely largely on manufacturers´ reports of physicochemical viscoelastic specifications and on company recommendations in their selection of a suitable agent. Manufacturer information is based on substance testing conducted by different institutes and sometimes reveals inconsistencies. The physicochemical characteristics must fulfill practical criteria which are essential for every-day operative use:

- Ease of injection
- Adequate protection of corneal endothelium and intraocular tissues
- Ability to occupy and maintain intraocular space
- Substance clarity (also during phacoemulsification)
- Ease of removal
- Low risk of postoperative intraocular pressure

We have attempted to reveal the actual conditions by running our own set of comparative tests in cooperation with the Max-Planck Institute for Polymer Research, Department of Rheology, Mainz, Germany.

Rheology is the study of the relationship between substance deformation and the forces generated by it. Ophthalmic viscosurgical devices (OVD) have both fluid and solid properties. Each substance has a specific distribution of physicochemical characteristics which define its clinical application.

Understanding this relationship allows us to select a specific substance to maintain the anterior chamber space, protect the corneal endothelium or coat instruments and tissues.

Viscoelastics are best described by the following terms:

- Viscosity
- Elasticity
- Viscoelasticity
- Pseudoplasticity
- Contact angle and surface tension (determine coatability)
- Rigidity
- Cohesiveness
- Temperature

To understand the mode of action of viscoelastic substance in ocular surgery, the following determinants are particularly important: viscosity, elasticity, viscoelasticity, pseudoplasticity and coatability.

Flow characteristics represent another way of describing viscoelastic properties involving rather complex models. Furthermore, variations are seen among manufacturers due to the use of individual techniques.

Flow Characteristics

Although flow mechanics are determined by their physical surroundings in more watery fluids, it is a substance's rheologic character which essentially determines flow characteristics among the more viscous and viscoelastic substances (Fig. 8).

Molecular reformation, following deformation by an external force, is time-dependent (Fig. 9). An external force exerted briefly and quickly, causes a viscoelastic substance to go out of shape for a short time only, allowing the substance to regain its shape as soon as the force is removed. If force is applied more slowly, the viscoelastic molecules gradually adapt to the new form. This relationship is easily seen in the following two models which also take into account the direction of the external force:

- pulling a heated, rolled dough bar quickly and forcefully on both ends would cause it to tear in the middle, resulting in two halves; pulling slowly on both ends causes the bar to elongate and become thinner.
- Moving a needle quickly through a high viscous viscoelastic substance would leave the needle standing at the point of insertion; moving a needle slowly through a high-viscous viscoelastic substance alters the shape of the viscoelastic mass and deforms it.

Basic rheologic terms should now be elucidated.

Viscosity

Viscosity describes the tendency of fluids to resist reciprocal laminar displacement of two adjacent layers: the so-called "inner friction". Viscosity is therefore a measure of fluid flow resistance. 1 % solutions of sodium hyaluronate (e.g., Healon® or Provisc®) show a viscosity 400,000 times higher than aqueous fluid. They are dependent on concentration, molecular weight, addition of solvent, and temperature. Viscosity can usually be determined by placing a certain amount of viscous fluid between two parallel plates of equal size at a predetermined distance from one another and sliding them in the same direction, at different speeds (Fig. 10).

The speed at which one plate is moved in relation to the other is called the shear rate, usually measured in radiant per second (rad/s) or in hertz (Hz, 1/s). The shear force, expressed in dynes/cm^2, is the force necessary per surface to displace the parallel-set plates. The velocity gradient is determined by the relative velocity of the plates divided by the fluid density. Dynamic viscosity is defined as the quotient of the shear force and the velocity gradient measured in $N \cdot sec \cdot m^{-2}$,

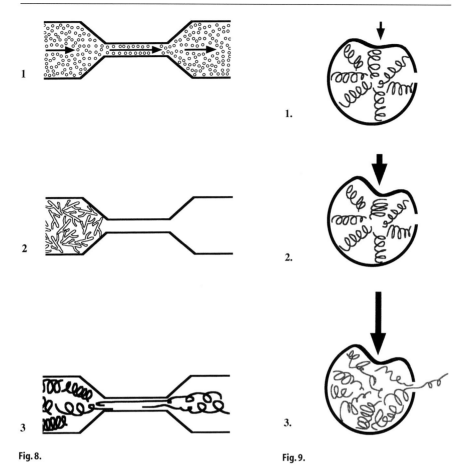

Fig. 8.   **Fig. 9.**

Fig. 8. Comparative diagram showing the flow behaviour of a waterlike, viscous, and viscoelastic fluid in a narrowing tube
1. waterlike substance: molecules flow faster through the narrow canal due to the fact that the same volume of fluid in a given time flows through a canal despite of the channels dimension
2. viscous substance: Here it depends on the ratio of the viscosity of the substance to the dimension of the canal if a certain viscous substance is able to pass through the narrowing tube
3. viscoelastic substance: The flowdrag of a viscoelastic substance will become lower depending on its movement. The chains of molecules are changing while passing the narrow canal. The flowdrag drops with the rising of the flow velocity because of the reorganised molecules. If there is enough space after the narrow passage the molecules are likely to change back to their original state

Fig. 9. Schematic picture showing the time and force-dependent behaviour of a viscoelastic substance. The viscoelastic substance is placed in a chamber with an opening
1. If a rather light force is applied for a short period of time the viscous properties of the substance will dominate
2. If a strong force is applied for a short time the substance will react elastic, in the way that the molecules will undergo deformation (without the chance of a reorganization). The force will be saved locally as elastic energy but none of the substance will leave the chamber
3. If a strong force is applied for a long period of time the phenomenon of shear stress will appear causing the molecules to change their shape. Then the flowdrag will become lower and therefore the substance will flow out of the chamber

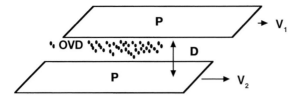

Fig. 10. Determination of viscosity: Two parallel plates of the same measure (P) are placed within a defined distance (D) from each other. They are moved in the same direction with different velocities(V_1, V_2). The fluid (OVD=ophthalmic viscosurgical device) is placed between the two plates

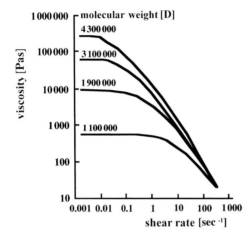

Fig. 11. The influence of the molecular weight on viscosity is shown as a function of the shear rate: A raise in molecular weight improves the viscosity with low shear rates. In the case of fairly high shear rates vicosity and molecular weight become independent from each other (modified according to Bothner and Wik, 1989)

Poise (P for Poiseuille). Kinetic viscosity represents the quotient of dynamic viscosity and fluid density (unit: Stokes, (St)).

The following relationships are noteworthy: viscosity is directly related to molecular weight and concentration, especially at low shear rates. However, it is inversely proportional to temperature (Fig. 11).

The viscosity at rest, i.e., zero shear rate, is clinically referred to as zero shear viscosity (unit: Pas = Pascal seconds = 1000 cp = 1000 centipoise). This value can not be accurately determined by a rheometer, but is rather extrapolated mathematically, using various computation methods. Viscosity at rest is occasionally employed as the single measure for the assessment and classification of behavioral properties of viscoelastic substances. However, viscosity at rest merely reflects one aspect of the varied biophysical characteristics of viscoelastic substances which merit differentiation.

The importance of viscosity at rest in ophthalmic surgery lies in the fact that viscoelastic fluids with a high viscosity value are particularly effective in deepening the anterior chamber, especially with raised vitreous pressure. Fluids with a very low value, such as irrigation solutions, require a constant flow to deepen the anterior chamber.

Influence of the Shear Rate on Viscosity

For use in ophthalmic surgery, knowing the viscosity at three different shear rates has proven to be helpful:
- Very low shear rates ($\sim 10^{-3}$ sec^{-1}) occur when ocular tissue is at rest and the viscoelastic substance occupies space during the operation.
- Medium shear rates ($\sim 10^{0}$ sec^{-1}) correspond approximately with the speed with which instruments are moved within the eye, or those occurring during IOL implantation.
- Very high shear rates ($\sim 10^{3}$ sec^{-1}) occur during viscoelastic substance injection through a cannula. Viscoelastic substances need very high viscosity at very low shear rates to maintain intraocular stability. Ophthalmic surgeons require low viscosity in order to move the IOL or instruments with the least possible resistance.

Elasticity

Elasticity, in the physical sense, describes the tendency of a substance to resist deformation and to regain its original shape again once the external force has been removed. Elasticity and viscosity are both a function of molecular weight and concentration. Substances with longer molecular chains typically show higher elastic properties. Elasticity is further dependent upon the frequency spectrum of the effecting force: sodium hyaluronate solutions behave as viscous fluids when mechanical energy in low-range frequency is applied, the polysaccharide chains unraveling under the force and forming a new molecular arrangement. Conversely, polysaccharide chains resist elastic deformation from high-range frequency mechanical energy. This implies that mechanical energy is stored in the form of elasticity and the solution behaves as an elastic body. In synovial fluid, vitreous humor or sodium hyaluronate solution, the transition from dominantly viscous characteristics to an elastic body occurs within the frequency range from 0.1 to 10 Hz. The viscoelastic properties of sodium hyaluronate have a shock absorbing as well as form stabilizing function in the tissues of the vitreous body, skin, joint cartilage and synovial fluid (Balazs & Gibbs, 1970).

Viscoelasticity

The term viscoelasticity itself named the substance group. Viscoelastic substances exert a minimal resistance to deformation, as opposed to elastic substances. They neither immediately regain their shape, nor does their shape restore completely (Hysteresis-effect, Fig.12). Viscoelastic substances have a relatively consistent form and do not regain their original shape following a deforming force, which differentiates them from plastic substances such as plasticine.

A viscoelastic substance behaves in both an elastic and viscous manner, as can best be described by the simplified mechanical model shown in Figure 13. The elastic element is represented by a coil and the viscous element by a plunger in oil (Bothner & Wik, 1989).

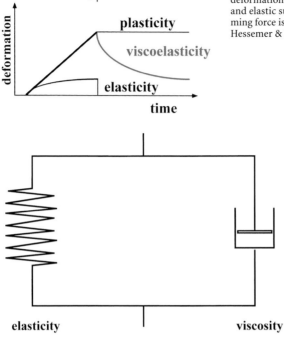

Fig. 12. Diagram showing the time-dependent deformation behaviour of plastic, viscoelastic, and elastic substances before and after a deforming force is applied (modified according to Hessemer & Dick, 1996)

Fig. 13. Mechanistic model to imitate the behaviour of a viscoelastic substance, combining elasticity and viscosity: The spring imitates the elastic behaviour which dominates if a force is brought upon the substance with a high frequency or high velocity. Meanwhile the piston represents the viscous flow behaviour at low frequencies

The response of this system depends on the speed of the effecting force and the oscillation frequency. At low speed or low frequencies, the flexible molecular network resembles a viscous solution. The energy applied is transformed into heat as the flexible molecules rub against each other. At high frequencies or quickly applied external force, the flexible molecular network is stretched, causing the viscoelastic to behave like a gel, elastically storing and then releasing most of the applied energy. High-molecular-weight hyaluronic acid behaves predominantly elastic at low shear rates, while low-molecular-weight hyaluronic acid behaves in a predominantly viscous manner. Increasing the concentration causes an increase in elastic components.

At low frequencies, viscous components prevail for all available viscoelastic substances used in ophthalmic surgery. With some viscoelastic substances, the elastic character increases and predominates with higher frequencies, while other solutions show mostly viscous properties at all frequencies.

Due to their relatively consistent form, viscoelastic substances are suitable as space-maintaining, surgical aids and, additionally, do not flow out of the anterior chamber easily following eye manipulation.

Pseudoplasticity

When viscosity is applied against the so-called speed-gradient, i.e., the relative speed of two plates moving in opposite directions or in like directions at different

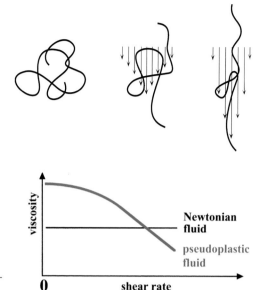

Fig. 14. The molecular arrangement depends on the movement. The molecule (hyaluronic acid) detangles as the shear rate rises (right)

Fig. 15. Diagram showing the coherence between viscosity and shear rate: The viscosity of viscoelastic substances declines with increasing velocity gradient (shear rate). This behaviour characterises pseudoelastic fluids

speeds, pseudoplastic fluids show a decrease in viscosity with an increasing gradient (Meaney, 1995). The reason for the high degree of pseudoplasticity of hyaluronic acid is the randomly coiled arrangement of the molecules at rest which increasingly uncoil with movement, thereby becoming less viscous (Fig. 14).

This pseudoplastic effect, i.e., the decrease in viscosity with increasing shear rate through untwining of hyaluronic acid molecules, is seen with intraocular injections of hyaluronic acid. The initially perceived resistance decreases substantially through the course of the injection (Fig. 15).

The pressure required to push the plunger down is directly proportional to the viscosity, underlining the necessity of a low viscosity at higher shear rates for injection through a thin cannula. By contrast, the viscosity of so-called Newtonian fluids, such as silicone oil or water, is independent of the shear rate. Pure chondroitin sulfate solutions or even hydroxypropylmethylcellulose solutions (according to a current school of thought) barely change (or not at all) their viscosity with increasing speed, defining them as Newtonian fluids.

The quotient of the viscosity at rest (zero shear viscosity) and the viscosity at a shear rate of 100/sec or 1000/sec is often used as a comparative measure for pseudoplasticity. This quotient alone gives an indication of the pseudoplastic potential of a fluid. However, the interpretation of this value at different shear rates is of importance. Pseudoplastic agents are of importance in ophthalmosurgery in so far as their high elasticity at rest provides good endothelial protection and possess space maintaining characteristics. Yet, they are easy to inject, aspirate and manipulate, and offer the advantage of staying in the eye longer during surgery, allowing protraction of their protective function.

Of all viscoelastic substances, sodium hyaluronate solution possesses the highest degree of pseudoplasticity. Pure chondroitin sulfate and HPMC solutions are regarded more as Newtonian fluids.

The reasons for the high pseudoplasticity of sodium hyaluronate are as follows: this high molecular polysaccharide is in an intertwined configuration at rest, forming a coil, so to speak (Fig. 16). These molecules, when brought into motion, "stretch" and become unraveled, resulting in a lowered viscosity (Gibbs et al., 1968). The course of the pseudoplasticity curve of a viscoelastic substance and the viscosity at speed gradient 0 are not only a function of the average molecular weight of the viscoelastic polymer, but also a function of the concentration. The viscosity at very high shear rates is, by contrast, independent of molecular weight.

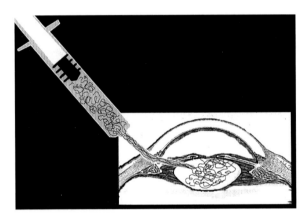

Fig. 16. Practical example to describe the behaviour of molecules of hyaluronic acids: In the syringe the molecules are entangled and interwined with each other. During injection the molecules detangle and pass the cannula unfolded. After the injection the molecules of the substance reorganise in the eye and change back to their primary conformation (as in the syringe). The viscosity is notably higher than during the passage through the cannula

At high shear rates, internal friction, and therefore, viscosity, are influenced primarily by the number of hyaluronic acid chains, since the molecules are stretched more and arranged lying along-side one another.

In summary, different viscoelastic substances have different viscosity and pseudoplasticity properties differentiating their use in intraocular surgery. A highly viscous sodium hyaluronate solution has excellent space maintaining qualities, lending itself suitably for anterior chamber deepening in cataract operations, especially with raised vitreous pressure. In contrast, a low viscosity chondroitin sulfate/sodium hyaluronate mixture, such as Viscoat®, has better surface related properties: the low pseudoplasticity of chondroitin sulfate is the contributing factor in its longer stay in the anterior segment, not being rinsed out so quickly, and thereby lending enduring protection to the corneal endothelium. This is of special interest in phacoemulsification, during which relatively high amounts of fluid volume per unit time pass over the eye, and in which corneal endothelial damage, in the form of air blisters, is a potential hazard. Furthermore, chondroitin sulfate possesses a strong affinity for and adhesion potential to PMMA and other IOL materials due to its strong negative charge (Hein, Keates & Weber, 1986). It is, therefore, especially useful for coating IOLs.

Coatability

The coating ability, i.e., the degree of adhesion of a viscoelastic substance, is determined by the angle formed between a fluid and a solid surface, and by surface tension. A viscoelastic substance creating a strong bulge on a surface reveals weak adhesion and a large contact angle is observed. A lesser contact angle and reduced surface tension indicate superior ability to wet and coat (Fig. 17). Viscoelastic agents with good wetting and coating capacities are good lubricants for instruments and syringes.

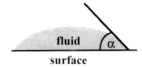

Fig. 17. Schematic picture showing the contact angle (α) with water, which has a significant influence on the ability of a substance to moisten a defined surface: the contact angle is formed by the angle between the adjacent surface and the water surface. There is an inverse proportionality between the moistening ability, the water contact angle, and the surface tension

Rigidity

The stiffness of a substance is calculated as the square root of the sum of the squares of viscosity and elasticity.

$$\sqrt{\text{viscosity}^2 + \text{elasticity}^2}$$

Cohesiveness

Cohesiveness describes the extent of intermolecular bonds or chains holding a substance together and is dependent on elasticity and molecular chain length. Long, high-molecular-weight chains of hyaluronate entwine in solution and lead to high cohesiveness. In an opened eye, a distortion of the bulb can cause the cohesive viscoelastic substance to leave the eye completely as a mass. Low-molecular viscoelastic substances have shorter, less interwoven chains and show a lower tendency to leave the eye as a mass. On the other hand, it is more difficult to aspirate such viscoelastics and therefore viscoelastic residue is sometimes found in the eye. This behavior is termed dispersive. Arshinoff (1997) introduced the so-called cohesive-dispersion index (CDI) as a clinical aid based on in-vitro exams of percentage removal of viscoelastic substance from the eye. The bigger the CDI (see below), measured by the percentage portion of aspirated OVD per unit time divided by the respective vacuum setting, the greater the cohesiveness of the OVD.

The CDIs of some popularly used viscoelastic substances are shown.

OVD	CDI (%/100 mmHg)
Healon® GV	77.3
Provisc®	46.0
Healon®	31.3
Amvisc® Plus	21.4
Viscoat®	3.4

Optical Properties of Viscoelastic Substances

Little is currently known about the optical properties of viscoelastic substances. Leith et al. (1987) reported on variable light absorption properties in the UV-range. Transparent fluids can be differentiated owing to the differing refractive indices of their surfaces. The refractive index is the most important property of a medium to refract light. A trial by Speicher & Göttinger showed only slightly different optical properties as related to temperature (25-42°C) and wavelength (479, 546, 643 nm) (Table 2).

All viscoelastic substances show a slightly higher refractive index than water.

Table 2. Refractive index of various viscoelastic substances (temperature 25°C; in decreasing order) modified according to Speicher & Göttinger, 1998

product	refractive index
Viscoat®	1.3446
AMO Vitrax®	1.3410
Hymecel®, Ocucoat®, Adatocel®, Methocel®	1.3390 to 1.3384
Amvisc® Plus, Healon® GV, Amvisc®, Dispasan®, Healon®	1.3382 to 1.3372
aqueous humor	1.336

Chemical Properties of Viscoelastic Substances, Biocompatibility and Safety Requirements

Specific safety requirements are placed on viscoelastic substances employed intraocularly. They must be sterile, pure and free of particles, as well as non-immunogenic, non-toxic and non-inflammatory. They must be biologically inert and show a balanced electrolyte content. Osmolality and colloid osmotic pressure as well as pH (see below) must correspond to corneal and aqueous humor values (pH = 7.38). They should be water-soluble and clear for implementation in the anterior chamber. Viscoelastic substances should be easily applied and removed, but, nonetheless, biologically transportable or biodegradable in the event of residues. They should be long-lasting and preferably storable at room temperature.

Content, molecular weight, pH-value, buffer substance and osmolality should all be included by the manufacturer in the product insert.

An overview of company information in terms of current commercially-marketed viscoelastic properties is presented in the Appendix Table. It is significant to take into account molecular weight, concentration and chemical composition when comparing these substances, especially with those manufactured by different companies.

Next to biological properties, the chemical characteristics of viscoelastic substances are key in their tolerability.

pH-Value

Although pH-values of currently available viscoelastic substances vary, manufacturers cite them at about the physiological norm of 7.38. Healon® and Viscoat® are supplied in a phosphate-buffered solution with a pH-range from 7.0 to 7.5 according to the manufacturers. Viscoat®, meanwhile, has a lower phosphate buffer concentration than originally, as higher phosphate concentration favors postoperative calcium precipitation in the corneal stroma with consecutive corneal epithelial clouding (Nevyas et al.,1987; Ullmann, Lichtenstein & Heerlein, 1986). This phenomenon was also observed after use of chondroitin sulfate alone. The pH-values of Amvisc® probably vary due to the addition of un-buffered physiological saline solution. The pH-value of HPMC solutions vary in accordance with their preparation, for instance, Ocucoat®, with a pH of almost 7.2 and Chiron Endocoat™, with a pH-value of 6.2, although companies generally claim pH-values do not reach far below 7.38 (see Appendix).

Colloid Osmotic Pressure

Both the osmotic and the colloid osmotic pressures are important when used in the human body, concerning biocompatibility of polymer solutions. The osmotic pressure is mostly influenced by the concentration of inorganic salts, while the colloid osmotic pressure is more dependent on concentration, polymer type, its molecular weight and the extent of interaction between the polymer molecules. In glycosaminoglycan-containing solutions, increasing concentrations quickly lead to an increase in the colloid osmotic pressure. The colloid osmotic pressure of hyaluronic acid is shown in Figure 18 as a function of concentration. Low molecular-weight solutions reach a physiologic colloid osmotic pressure of 30 mmHg at concentrations of 10 mg/ml, while high molecular-weight solutions reach the same pressure at concentrations of 15 mg/ml. Similar curves were

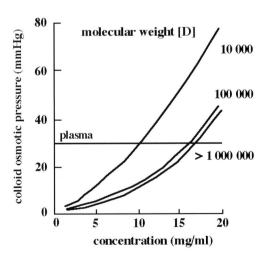

Fig. 18. Dependency of the colloid osmotic pressure of hyaluronate on the concentration and the molecular weight (modified according to Bothner & Wik, 1989)

described for chondroitin sulfate containing solutions (Shaw, 1976). Yielding of a solution with colloid osmotic pressure above the physiological level leads to dehydration of cells and tissues as reported by Hedby (1963).

Osmolality

The osmolality of a solution describes the amount of unbound particles per 1 kg water in Mol (Osmol/kg H_2O). The higher the osmolality of a viscoelastic substance with respect to the intercellular fluid, which is about 300 milliosmol per kg, the greater its potential to dehydrate adjacent tissues. Chondroitin sulfate, at concentrations of 20 and 50%, shows extremely high osmolality, in both chemical laboratory examinations and clinical experience (Condon et al., 1983). In contrast, osmolarity describes the amount of unbound particles per liter solution in Mol (Osmol/l). Aqueous humor has an osmolality of 305 milliosmol. Human corneal endothelium tolerates fluids with osmolality between 200-400 milliosmol and experiences endothelial cell damage with fluids of low osmolality (Hyndiuk & Schulz, 1992). The single-celled-layer of healthy corneal endothelium exposed to hypo-osmotic fluid (240 mOsm) swells, due to the osmotic gradient. Gap and tight junctions are not compromised, however, nor is any long-term damage observed (McDermott et al., 1988). Corneas with low endothelial cell-count (less than 1000 cells/mm^2) or functional disturbances are seen to experience, in addition to intracellular edema, the breaking of intercellular bridges with the consecutive flowing in of fluids into the corneal stroma, with ensuing corneal edema (Gonnering et al., 1979). The cornea consequently swells (Fig. 19).

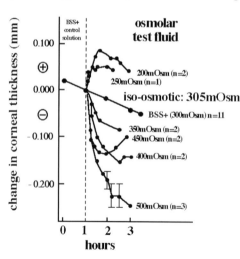

Fig. 19. Time-dependent influence of hypo- and hyperosmotic BSS solution on the thickness of the human cornea (modified according to Edelhauser et al., 1981)

Structural Formulas and Chemical Composition

Chondroitin sulfate and sodium hyaluronate share similar chemical and physical characteristics. They consist of repeating disaccharide sub-units: sodium glucuronate in β 1-3 linkage with N-acetylgalactosamine for sodium chondroitin sulfate (Fig. 20), and N-acetylglucosamine for sodium hyaluronate (Fig. 21). The sub-units are then combined by β 1-4 linkage of the amino sugar residue to the glucu-ronic residue of the next sub-unit to form large polymers. Both chains occur as a large, unbranched chain structure of medium to high molecular weight (Meyer, 1958). The two compounds differ in that sodium chondroitin sulfate possesses a sulfate group and a double, rather than a single, negative charge (as is the case with sodium hyaluronate), per repeating disaccharide sub-unit (Fig. 20). The ad-ditional negative charge per chondroitin sulfate sub-unit has a neutralizing effect on tissues, implants and instruments which are positively charged. This chemical property will possibly explain the good coating capacity of chondroitin sulfate, specifically Viscoat®.

The binding of medication to the viscoelastic substance in the eye seems to be of secondary importance in the cases of Amvisc®, Healon®, and Viscoat®. Visco-elastics, thus, have no absorptive mechanism influencing the effects of intraocu-lar or topical therapeutics (McDermott & Edelhauser, 1989).

Cellulose, a disaccharide of D-glucose, represents the basic molecule, stereo-chemically differing from dextrose in the bonds existing between the two mono-mers: a β-glycoside bond in cellulose and a α-glycoside bond in dextrose. To in-crease hydrophilic properties, methoxy- and hydroxypropyl- side-chains are re-placed by hydroxy groups (Fig. 22). The molecule is uncharged.

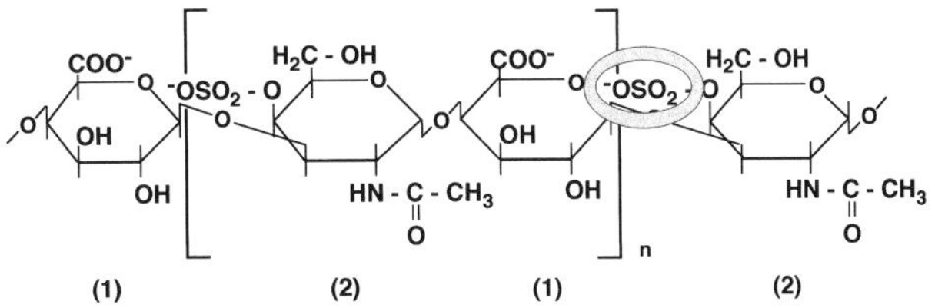

Fig. 20. Chemical structure formula of the bisaccharinic portion of chondroitin-4-sulfate, a proteogly-can, consisting of a repetitive basic unit made of D-glucuronic acid (1) and N-acetyl-D-galactosamine-4-sulfate (2). The glycosidic bonds are alternating β 1-3 and β 1-4 bonded. The additional negative charge per sub-unit (circled) gives the molecule a high density of charge

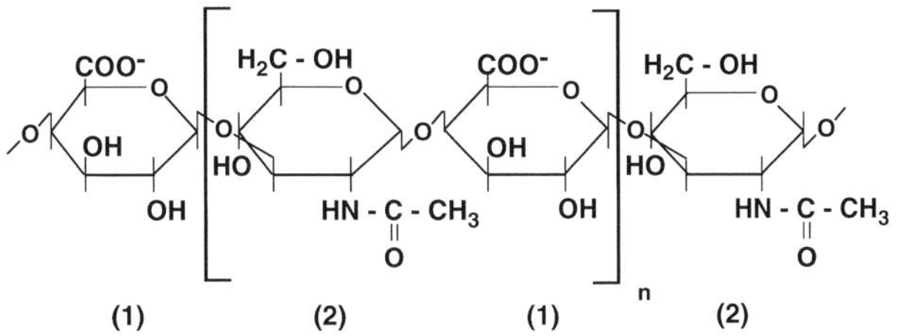

Fig. 21. Chemical structure formula of the hyaluronic acid, consisting of a repetitive basic unit made up by β-D-glucuronic acid (1) and N-acetyl-β-D-galactosamine (2). The glycosidic bonds are alternating β 1-3 and β 1-4 bonded. The molecular formula of the linear polymeric sodium hyaluronic acid reads as follows: $(C_{14}H_{20}NNaO_{11})_n$

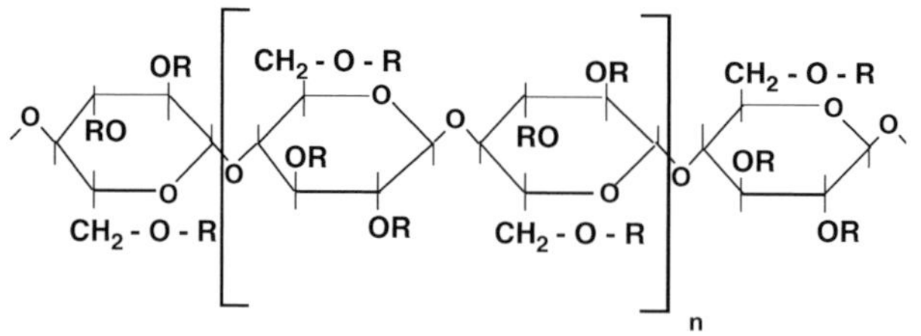

OR | CH₂-O-R | OR | CH₂-O-R

(chemical structure diagram)

Fig. 22. Chemical structure formula of hydroxypropylmethylcellulose. The monomeric units of the polysaccharide are connected with each other through β-glycosidic bonds
R=H,
  CH₃ or
  CH₂-CH(OH)-CH₃

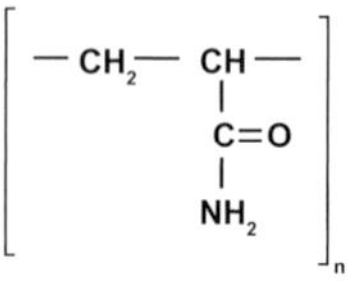

$$-CH_2-CH-\\ \quad | \\ \quad C=O \\ \quad | \\ \quad NH_2$$

Fig. 23. Chemical structure formula of polyacrylamide (Orcolon®), polymeric acrylamide, consisting of long atomic chains of carbon

The structural formula of polyacrylamide is represented in Figure 23.

Within the sodium hyaluronate molecule, reduced flexibility at the glycoside bond causes a rotation of carbohydrate units along the molecule chain. As a consequence, the molecule shows a flexible, random coil conformation with a certain rigidity. Chondroitin sulfate, however, is a low-molecular-weight glycosaminoglycan and assumes a conformation between the coil described above and a rigid rod.

Sodium hyaluronate contains no other carbohydrates or amino acids and shows no covalent intermolecular bonds (Balazs, 1983). In such solutions as water or aqueous, this rigid molecule takes on the form of a very flexible and long random coil. Small molecules can penetrate into and disperse inside the sodium hyaluronate molecule, while larger molecules, such as fibrinogen, collagen or proteoglycan, cannot (Balazs, 1983). Osmotic activity, as well as, the interaction of molecules in the intercellular matrix, have often been pointed out as the influence of this so-called steric exclusion of transport (Comper & Laurent, 1978).

An increase in the sodium hyaluronate concentration of a solution causes an overlapping of individual molecular coils, as well as, a compression (Fig. 24).

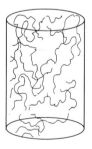 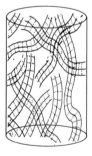

Fig. 24. Different concentrations of sodium hyaluronate in a cylindrical device: left hand side low concentrated and right hand side higher concentrated hyaluronic acid. In a solvent the chains of the hyaluronic acid are slightly tangled (left). Meanwhile in a higher concentrated solution (right) a compression of the tangled chains takes place. This close proximity of the molecular chains leads to different, non-covalent interactions between the chains and causes an increase of viscosity and elasticity of the solution

Furthermore, non-covalent side-chain interaction increases. Following sodium hyaluronate injection into the anterior chamber and during its presence there, molecular size changes only slightly. This suggests that neither oxidation nor enzymatic degradation play a large role in its breakdown. Thus, sodium hyaluronate is not metabolized in the eye, but rather passes through the trabecular meshwork in large molecular form. Its break down in the anterior chamber largely depends upon viscosity and injected amount (Miyauchi & Iwata, 1984). HPMC, on the other hand, experiences partial metabolism before leaving the eye.

All polymers usually contain molecules of varying molecular weight. The manufacturer commonly lists the average molecular weight value. The size of sodium hyaluronate set for production varies. Amvisc®, for example, is formulated to a molecular weight of 2 million Daltons, a dynamic viscosity of 40 000 mPas at 25°C and a shear rate of 2 per second. Healon®, in contrast, is formulated to a concentration of 10 mg/ml (compare to information leaflet).

Chondroitin sulfate in Viscoat® has a mean molecular weight of 22 500 D, while sodium hyaluronate in Viscoat® has a mean molecular weight of over 500 000 D. The combined molecular weight of Viscoat® has a value of somewhere less than 600 000 D. The manufacturer avers that the short molecular chains of Viscoat® pass through the trabecular meshwork and, hence, leave the eye more easily.

Complications through Viscoelastics

Problems of diverse nature have been observed ever since the first applications of viscoelastics to the present day (Table 3). All currently approved viscoelastics cause an increase in intraocular pressure, especially in the early, postoperative phase (Cherfan, Rich & Wright; Holmberg & Philipson, 1984a and 1984b). In early applications, band-shaped keratopathy, corneal dehydration or contaminations were at times observed following injections of highly concentrated chondroitin sulfate solution. Orcolon® was taken off the market due to incidences of late, secondary glaucoma (Herrington, Ball & Updegraf, 1993). In the beginning phases of production of Viscoat, the product was temporarily removed from the market as a result of endotoxins and calcium chelate formation in the anterior stroma portion of the cornea due to the addition of phosphate-buffer (Coffman & Mann,

Table 3. Overview of problems and complications after the use of viscoelastic substances in the past

problem/complication	product	year
increase in IOP	Healon®	1980
band keratopathy	Viscoat®	1984
corneal dehydration	chondroitin sulfate	1986
contamination	Viscoat®	1988
sterility	Ocucoat®	1991
late secondary glaucoma	Orcolon®	1991
contamination	Microvisc®	1993
crystalline IOL deposits	Healon® GV	1994
sterile uveitis	Dispasan®	1997
endotoxin content (100 EU/ml)	Microvisc®	1997

1986; Binder, Deg & Kohl, 1987; Nevyas et al., 1987). Both problems have been resolved by the manufacturer and not repeated since.

In recent years, use of Microvisc® and Dispasan® (Grisanti et al., 1997) revealed pseudoendophthalmitis-like reactions. In an eye-clinic in Montreal, Canada, a series of 14 cases of endophthalmitis appeared, most of which proved to be caused by bacterial contamination (Bacillus circulans) of the viscoelastic product applied (Microvisc® Company: Q-med AB, Uppsala, Sweden, two separate batches) in 1993 following a total of 42 ophthalmosurgeries performed (Roy et al., 1997). The company, Bohus BioTech AB, Strömstad, Sweden, bought the product name Microvisc® for its viscoelastic in 1995, 2 years following the above-mentioned contamination of a viscoelastic of the same name. In the case of Microvisc® (once more available in Germany unchanged, as opposed to its availability in several other countries), a higher endotoxin content of over 100 U/ml was discovered in 1997, while a maximum content of 0.5 Units is recommended (Florén, Hansen & Ehringer, 1997). Florén reports that in January, 1997, in Oslo, Norway, three suspected pseudoendophthalmitis-like reactions were observed following cataract surgery. Similar observations had also been made at other Swedish and Norwegian hospitals after use of this particular batch of viscoelastic. At the University Eye-Clinic Lund, an endophthalmitis-like anterior chamber reaction with flaky precipitation in a coagulated exudate was seen one day following a combined operation in which Microvisc® residues were left in the anterior chamber of one eye. Following intensive antiphlogistic therapy without beneficial effects on the anterior chamber, Microvisc® was surgically removed from the anterior chamber 24 hours postoperatively (Florén, 1998). The Norwegian batch mentioned earlier, as well as other batches, were contaminated by endotoxin with up to 100 U/ml, according to reports made by Florén (Florén, Hansen & Ehringer, 1997). An intraocular inflammatory response with the consequent development of bullous keratopathy was described in a series of cases after use of Healon® which was spread by the implementation of a reused injection cannula (Nuyts et al., 1990). Manufacturers now supply single-use cannulas along with each batch of viscoelastic. It was suggested that reuse of cannulas be avoided, as this was seen to promote corneal edema (Hyndiuk & Schulz, 1992; Kim, 1987).

Healon® GV was associated with crystalline deposits on the IOL, which remained there for a temporary period of time, and the cause of which was not clarified by the authors (Jensen et al., 1994). These complications were not substantiated by any other authors.

The suspicion that HPMC application in cataract surgery lead to long-lasting pupillary dilation (Eason & Seward, 1995) was not proven. A comparison between Healon® and Ocucoat® showed no difference in pupillary width and reactivity 6 months postoperatively.

Unfortunately, contaminations occur throughout the history of viscoelastics (compare Table 3). Manufacturers are hopefully taking precautions to preclude future incidences of OVD contamination.

Both laboratory and clinical examinations confirm that Healon®, Viscoat® and many other viscoelastics have no inflammatory effects when produced in the proper combinations. Specific tests (such as the owl monkey eye test) carried out prior to the release of a batch of hyaluronic acid confirm this finding in Healon®, Healon®5 and Healon® GV (see below). For HPMC products, implantation tests in the anterior chamber of rabbit eyes were performed to test for biological tolerance (Becker et al., 1988; Ehrich, 1987; Ehrich, Höh & Kreiner, 1990).

Allergic reactions, as unwanted side-effects of viscoelastic use, are theoretically possible, but quite rare (Glasser et al., 1991).

The Owl Monkey Eye Test

A highly sensitive test is required for the detection of endotoxic inflammatory substances to evaluate the purity of sodium hyaluronate. The Limulus-Lysate-Test, a highly sensitive test for pyrogens, was observed to be neither sensitive nor specific enough to detect impurities in sodium hyaluronate solutions.

Examination procedures for the detection of cell-mediated inflammatory reactions in tissue compartments (e.g., anterior chamber, peritoneum, joint spaces) were also deemed not sensitive enough to detect this particular type of reaction mediator.

Owl- and rhesus-monkey eyes reveal the presence of minute amounts of endotoxin introduced into the relatively large amount of aqueous humor volume along with physiological buffers. The vitreous humor of these monkey eyes is fluid and can be exchanged for test-solution with relatively little surgical trauma.

The adult rhesus monkey offers only limited assistance in detecting endotoxins, as the potential volume exchange of its fluid vitreous is around 0.4-0.6 ml, and the rest of the vitreous volume comprises 2.4 ml in the form of formed vitreous body. In contrast to this, an exchange volume of 2 ml fluid vitreous is available in the adult owl monkey eye (Fig. 25). The greater the amount of fluid exchange volume, the greater also the amount of injectable test fluid. Forty-eight hours following the intravitreal injection of test solution, anterior chamber paracentesis is performed, with consequent sequestering of aqueous humor to quantify the induced inflammatory reaction. The sequestered aqueous humor is useful in counting leukocytes as well as determining protein concentration and protein distribution among other things. As a reference, a similar volume of buffer solution is exchanged (instead of sodium hyaluronate solution).

Fig. 25. Owl-faced guenun

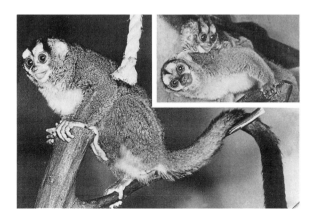

Forty-eight hours following the intravitreal injection of test solution, the average leukocyte count in aqueous humor should be 28 ± 7 cells/mm^3, and protein content should be 10.8 ± 2.8 mg/ml, after exchange of 1 ml fluid vitreous against the same volume of sterile, pyrogen-free, physiological buffer solution under sterile conditions and with minimal surgical trauma.

Sodium hyaluronate solution, as well as any other fluid used in intraocular surgery, should evoke a low inflammatory reaction to the vitreous body, similar to that of physiological buffer solution, under like test conditions.

International Organization for Standardization

Several years ago, a working group was formed (ISO, International Organization for Standardization) with the intention of elaborating an acceptable, world-wide standard for OVD preparation, registration and manufacturer information leaflets. The ISO is concerned with the implementation of viscoelastics as 'medicinal products', which, however, do not have (at least seen with some manufacturers) the comparable sterilization procedures required of drugs. Sterilization by autoclave is not performed due to partial sodium hyaluronic acid degradation, which would forfeit its rheologic properties to a certain extent. Some companies perform a terminal sterilization by autoclave to sterilize their products. Other companies aseptically filter their products, a process by which, however, a much lower degree of sterilization is achieved. The ISO-working-group is striving to encourage manufacturers to print the degree of product sterilization on the package.

CHAPTER 3

Viscoelastic Substances

Hyaluronate

Hyaluronate (Fig. 26) is found in almost all vertebrate connective tissues, and consists of a relatively long, linear polysaccharide molecule (Balazs, et al., 1970). It is synthesized in the cell membrane and the long, linear polysaccharide chain is extruded directly into the extracellular matrix (Prehm, 1984). Sodium hyaluronate serves to stabilize cells and tissues and plays an important role during embryonic development and growth. On the cellular level, sodium hyaluronate is involved in intercellular interactions, cell matrix adhesions, cell mobility and extracellular organization. It also accelerates wound healing (Abatangelo, Martelli & Vecchia, 1983; Arzeno & Miller, 1982) and seems to function as a natural biological substance.

In the eye, high concentrations of sodium hyaluronate are present in the vitreous humor and in the connective tissue of the trabecular chamber angle. It is found in aqueous humor, although only in low concentrations, and covers the endothelium. Human corneal endothelial cells retain specific binding-sites for hyaluronic acid (Härfstrand et al., 1992). The normal human eye has a hyaluronic acid concentration of 1.4 mg/l (Laurent & Laurent, 1981), which covers the corneal endothelium in a thin, uninterrupted coat (Fig. 27), the function of which has not yet been clarified. The hyaluronic acid endothelial coating is presumably involved in

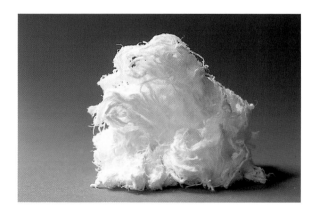

Fig. 26. Purified hyaluronic acid, obtained from the roosters comb

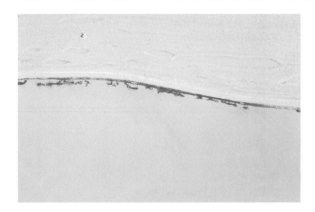

Fig. 27. Histologic cut through the human cornea after staining the bound hyaluronic acid with the help of the Avidinperoxidase-method: The surface of the corneal endothelium shows a thin but dense colour after streptomyces-hyaluronidase treatment to ensure the specificity of the staining method in the first place. Hyaluronic acid had been injected into the anterior chamber 5 minutes prior to this treatment and was followed by an irrigation-/aspiration maneuvre with 100 ml BSS (light microscopy)

the regulation of tissue hydration and transendothelial transport of macromolecules. After anterior chamber hyaluronic acid injection and subsequent implementation of hyaluronic acid detection methods, the thickness and color intensity of the hyaluronic acid coat were seen to have increased. Single endothelial cells show approximately 2000 binding-sites (Madsen et al., 1989), which presumably have a higher affinity for high molecular weight hyaluronic acid. There is both skepticism and support among ophthalmosurgeons as to whether the receptor-bound hyaluronic acid coat continues to lend further endothelial-cell protection against surgically-induced traumas once hyaluronic acid has been extensively removed from the eye (Schmidl, Mester & Anterist, 1998).

Sodium hyaluronate plays a role in controlling aqueous flow in the trabecular meshwork.

This substance is also a constituent of the streptococcal capsule and is one of the few polysaccharides present in bacteria.

The molecular weight of hyaluronate, as derived from different sources, is within the range of $0.1 \times 10^6 - 10 \times 10^6$ D (Laurent & Granath, 1983). Sodium hyaluronate is part of the glycosaminoglycan group, constituting a large polyanionic polysaccharide molecule containing hexosamine. All other vertebrate glycosaminoglycans distinguish themselves from hyaluronate in the following three points: low molecular weight (10 000-40 000 D), covalent protein binding (proteoglycans) and covalent sulfesther-group binding (chondroitin sulfate, keratan sulfate, dermatan sulfate, heparan sulfate, heparin). Chondroitin, a non-sulfated variant of chondroitin sulfate, constitutes the only exception.

A single molecule comprises a spherically shaped space of 0.5 μm in diameter. High-molecular hyaluronic acid, in solution, does not exist in the form of a long, rigid and straight chain. The polysaccharide glycoside linkages allow a rotation of the carbohydrate units along the molecule chain, restricting hyaluronate flexibility. The result is a coil-like configuration with rigid characteristics (Laurent, 1957). The spacial stretching of the coil is determined by the type of glycoside bonds present, the existence of large side chains, the polyelectrolytic character and probably also the distribution of intermolecular hydrogen bonds. The linear hyaluronic acid polysaccharide, with a molecular weight of 4×10^6 D, is made out of approximately 10 000 disaccharid units, with an average molecular chain diameter of

300 nm, a chain length of 10 000 nm and a volume of about 10 nl in solution. Lowering the molecular weight leads to a more rigid conformation of the hyaluronic acid molecule (Laurent, 1957).

Hyaluronate, which shows a serum half-life of 4 minutes, is only slightly metabolized in the eye and is predominantly catabolized by hepatic endothelial cells (Fraser et al., 1981; Laurent & Fraser, 1990; Laurent, Dahl & Lilja, 1993). The origin of hyaluronic acid (rooster combs, biofermentation) hardly seems to have an influence here (Nimrod et al.,1992).

Balazs suggested the implementation of sodium hyaluronate for vitreous replacement in retinal detachment surgery after working for over 20 years in researching the molecular structure and biological behavior of endocellular matrix polysaccharides. As little was known at the time about the pathophysiology of the vitreous body or about retinal detachment, the use of sodium hyaluronate was not properly implemented and soon abandoned. Miller and coworkers (1977) were the first to again renew interest in this substance, as IOL implantations became more wide-spread. Balazs patented a highly purified form of sodium hyaluronate and published a report on its uses within the context of intraocular surgery (1979).

The manufacturers of sodium hyaluronate stress the importance of substance purity. Many manufacturers have their own methods to achieve this high quality. Numerous sources are known to harbor sodium hyaluronate: rooster combs, umbilical cord or streptococcal cultures (Fig. 28).

Ultrapurified forms of sodium hyaluronate from these different sources always retain the same structure. The molecular weight can vary considerably, changing the physical characteristics and, therefore, representing a considerable influence.

A special production process was developed for the production of sodium hyaluronate through microbial fermentation with streptococci. It is possible to produce different sodium hyaluronates with varying molecular weights for diverse pharmaceutical and cosmetic applications. The company, Fermentech (London, England), for instance, produces sodium hyaluronate in this manner. The process employed, however, is continuous, as opposed to the otherwise standard production of individual batches. In batch cultures, cells are found at varying stages of the cell cycle, and therefore, at different metabolic states. That is to say, some or-

Fig. 28. A roosters head with comb from which hyaluronic acid can be extracted

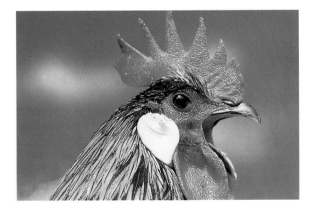

ganisms produce sodium hyaluronate, while others break it down. The result is a high cell wall turn-over, with unwanted metabolic products, such as diverse acids. With continuous fermentation, the cell wall turn-over is minimized and it is possible, through a targeted alteration of growth conditions in the culture, to produce sodium hyaluronate with different molecular weights. There is controversy as to whether sodium hyaluronate is more consistent and less proteinaceous as derived from rooster combs or from bacterial fermentation.

The first commercially available sodium hyaluronate was Healon®. It was sold by Balazs, who owned the rights, to Pharmacia (Uppsala, Sweden), and was subsequently developed by the company Biomatrix. Healon® was introduced in 1980. Certain sodium hyaluronate effects can be explained by the influence of certain cell functions, such as: inhibition of in-vitro migration of granulocytes, macrophages and lymphocytes; inhibition of phagocytotic activity of macrophages and granulocytes; inhibition of prostaglandin release and inhibition of lymphocyte transformation, such as in-vitro inhibition of vascular endothelial cell growth (Balazs, 1983; Balazs, 1986). Soon other rooster comb hyaluronic acid viscoelastics came on the market, such as Amvisc®, differing from Healon® in few aspects only. Healon® has a different buffer solution and a different UV-light absorption spectrum in the range of 230-330 nm, which makes the existence of similar biological substances likely (Leith et al., 1987).

Every sodium hyaluronate solution harbors a certain inflammatory potential which varies from batch to batch (McKnight, Giagiacomo & Adelstein, 1987). It is independent of its origin, concentration or constitution (Hultsch, 1980). This inflammatory potential is best determined by an intravitreal injection into the owl monkey eye, followed by a slit lamp examination of the inflammatory process in the anterior chamber and vitreous body. This process has been established as a reproducible biological examination.

Autoclaving of sodium hyaluronate results in a significant depolymerization and change in viscosity (see below; Kim, 1987). Responsible for the relatively high expense associated with sodium hyaluronate solution are the considerable, technological demands for the production of a non-inflammatory compound, at a predetermined molecular weight.

Sodium hyaluronate solutions, except AMO®, Vitrax® and Rayvisc®, must be stored in cool storage places to preserve their physicochemical properties.

Hydroxypropylmethylcellulose

Methyl cellulose is widely distributed in nature, as seen in cotton and wood, although not in humans or animals.

Hydroxypropylmethylcellulose (HPMC) is synthesized from methylcellulose.

A 1% methylcellulose solution was described first by Fechner (1977) for IOL coating just prior to implantation in cataract surgery. A 2% solution was better suited, in contrast to the 1% solution, for space maintaining purposes (Fechner, 1983). In ophthalmology, methylcellulose is used as a lubricant and contact gel, e.g., for contact glass examinations, as well as the long-known foundation used in eye-drops. Highly purified HPMC is composed of long glucose chains, whose hydroxy group is replaced up to 29 % by methoxypropyl side-chains and up to 8.5% by hydroxypropyl side-chains. This side-chain substitution renders HPMC more hydrophilic than pure methylcellulose. Fechner described a method for the purification of HPMC, which was slightly modified later (Fechner, 1977; Fechner, 1985). Today there is a wide variety of HPMC products of varying concentrations and molecular weights (compare Appendix). In the US, HPMC was first commercially produced by Barnes & Hinde and licensed by the FDA.

Many HPMC products, like Ocucoat®, are primarily sold as viscoadherents, and less as real viscoelastic substances. Their wetting and coating capacities are highlighted against a background of several other positive viscoelastic properties due to the comparatively small contact angle and low surface tension. A multitude of experiments ascertain HPMC as a safe and effective viscoelastic substance for application in cataract operations with IOLs , in both animals and humans (Aaron-Rosa et al., 1983; Baba, Kasahara & Momose, 1987; Bigar et al., 1988; Kerr Muir et al., 1987; Liesegang, Bourne & Ilstrup, 1986; MacRae et al., 1983; Smith et al., 1984; Steele, 1989; Thompsen, Simonsen & Andreassen, 1987). HPMC, however, does not exist in animals or humans, and therefore, is not physiological. It is not completely metabolized in the anterior chamber of the eye and its metabolism beyond the trabecular meshwork is not well known.

HPMC is eliminated from the anterior chamber of rabbit eyes within 48 hours, independent of molecular weight, concentration or viscosity (Ehrich, Höh & Kreiner, 1990). An enzymatic digestion of HPMC is, however, only alluded to (Fernandez-Vigo, Refojo & Jumblatt, 1989). HPMC evoked serious inflammatory reactions after application in the vitreous body in animal experiments, dependent on which preparation was applied (Koster & Sztilma, 1986). The different mixtures produced by individual hospital pharmacies contain diverse solid parts (Rosen & Gregory, 1989). These are predominantly plant fibers from the original material and remain part of the end-product regardless of preparation (Kwitko & Belfort, 1991; Rosen, Gregory & Barnett, 1986). The explanation for this lies in the fact that HPMC solubility is dependent on temperature. Aggregated HPMC, which assumes a gel form, makes the production of a particle-free intraocular solution difficult. Furthermore, crystalline complexes form with relative ease in solution. Both aggregation and crystalline complex formation are resolvable within the context of commercial production with appropriate filtering processes. Unfortunately, no guidelines currently exist for HPMC-production purity for intraocular use, such as the purity criteria of the Union of German Pharmacists. An eye ointment sample (10 µg) examined is to contain no more than 20 particles larger than 25 µm, maximally 2 particles larger than 50 µm and no particles exceeding 90 µm.

HPMC is usually sterilized by autoclave, which is to its advantage, as opposed to other viscoelastics, because it remains unchanged by the autoclave process. HPMC does, nonetheless, have a tendency for microbial contamination, which is why special attention is given to filtering processes post-autoclave to ensure endo- and exotoxin removal from the substance. Quality control is of particular relevance here since HPMC products retain precipitates. More advantages of HPMC are: storage at room temperature, availability and low HPMC production-costs. The necessary biotechnical purification-processes are, however, costly. Hydroxypropylmethylcellulose lasts 3 years, at room temperature.

Chondroitin Sulfate

Chondroitin sulfate is a constituent of human extracellular matrix. It is the main polysaccharide component found in solid tissue-parts like cartilage, unlike sodium hyaluronate, which is found mostly in soft tissues like aqueous and vitreous fluids, and synovial membranes. The cornea has the highest concentration of chondroitin sulfate. Chondroitin sulfate, like sodium hyaluronate, is a polysaccharide and is predominantly extracted from shark-fin cartilage. During biosynthesis, carbohydrate units bind to the protein chain. Chondroitin sulfate does not exist as a free polysaccharide in nature, but rather as a constituent of protein-polysaccharide molecules, called proteoglycans. In contrast to sodium hyaluronate, chondroitin sulfate contains sulfur groups which have a double negative charge. This negative charge, per repeated chondroitin sulfate unit, is responsible for the high degree of adherence to positively charged tissue parts. The coating of IOL surfaces with chondroitin sulfate leads to a reduction of electrostatic interaction between the IOL and the endothelium (Harrison et al., 1982). The molecular weight of chondroitin sulfate is 20000 D (Table 4). It has a short chain length of approximately 50 nm, contrasted to sodium hyaluronate chain length of about 10000 nm (Bothner & Wik, 1983).

Due to the low viscosity at rest, a 20% solution of chondroitin sulfate is a useful agent in tissue coating (Soll et al., 1980) and a less instrumental agent in space retention or tissue separation. Increasing the concentration and viscosity (e.g. 50% chondroitin sulfate) leads to hyperosmosis and endothelial dehydration with cell damage (MacRae et al., 1983; Soll et al., 1980). Viscoat® is a 1:3 mixture of 4% chondroitin sulfate and 3% sodium hyaluronate. The sodium hyaluronate in Viscoat® is derived from bacterial fermentation using a gene technology production sequence. The chondroitin sulfate in Viscoat® is extracted from shark-fin cartilage. The mixture of the substances enhances the positive characteristics of each, i.e., high viscosity and space effectiveness of sodium hyaluronate, as well as, coating ability and cell protective effects of chondroitin sulfate.

Table 4. Comparison of the number of disaccharid units, molecular weight and chain length in hyaluronic acid and chondroitin sulfate

substance	units (n =)	molecular weight (D)	chain length (nm)
disaccharid unit	1	400	1
chondroitin sulfate	50	20 000	50
hyaluronic acid			
low molecular weight	1 000	400 000	1 000
high molecular weight	10 000	4 000 000	10 000

Polyacrylamide

Polyacrylamide (Orcolon®) is mentioned primarily out of historical interest. It was produced by Optical Radiation Cooperation (ORC, Azusa, California, USA) as a purely synthetic substance composed of polyacrylamide, a polymer of acrylamide, and was used for years in electrophoresis and chromatography. It is made out of long carbon chains, such as seen in fatty acids or carotenes, and does not need to be stored at cool temperatures.

Orcolon® leaves the eye after a few short hours. It is, however, broken down and eliminated by the liver and spleen after several weeks. In the hopes of increasing viscosity, several different ingredients were added to it. Polyacrylamide has a small contact angle, which enhances its coating capacity. Initial trials on rabbits and monkeys proved polyacrylamide as safe and comparable to 1% sodium hyaluronate with respect to intraocular pressure development and postoperative biomicroscopic as well as scanning electron microscopic endothelial findings (Roberts & Pfeiffer, 1989). Based on these results, it was applied in cataract surgery. In a randomized comparison to Healon®, no statistically significant differences were observed within a 3 month span following ECCE, with regard to postoperative intraocular pressure and endothelial cell loss (Mortimer, Sutton & Henderson, 1991). There were, however, several cases of late secondary glaucoma following use of polyacrylamide and it was subsequently removed from the market by its manufacturers (Herrington, Ball & Updegraff, 1993; Siegel et al., 1991). The probable cause is considered to be netting polyacrylamide (so-called microgel), which accumulates in the canal of Schlemm and in the trabecular meshwork (as seen in cows, monkeys and humans), leading to late, postoperative increases in intraocular pressure (Kaufman et al., 1994).

Collagen

Human placental collagen type 4 seems to be a useful viscoelastic substance (Charleux et al., 1987). Collagen is a protein found in the human basal membrane. All other viscoelastic substances are polysaccharides. Several different collagen preparations are produced, based on temperature, pH-value and ionic composition (Bothner & Wik, 1989). To the present day, very little information is available as to the best source of collagen, or as to the best type of collagen for intraocular surgery. Collagen type 4 has no visible fibrils, as opposed to types I-III, which makes it suitable for production of transparent fluid. The commercial product is sold under the name Collagel® and has a molecular weight of over 1 million D. There are, however, complications associated with the use of proteins intraocularly (Balazs, 1989). Human collagen (Collagel®) has been evaluated in very few clinical trials (Charleux et al., 1987; Charleux et al., 1989). Leckmann and coworkers (1992) found no statistically significant differences in comparing Collagel® with Healon® in 48 eyes undergoing cataract operation with IOL implantation with regards to intraocular pressure, corneal thickness, endothelial cell loss and visual acuity. Pork collagen is employed as an implant to improve the results of deep sclerectomies (Fa. STAAR Surgical, Monrovia, California, USA).

Cellugel®

The viscoelastic Cellugel® is composed of a synthetic polymer-modified carbohydrate, formulated to a molecular weight of approximately 100 000 D and a viscosity between 12-15 000 cps at 25 °C. It can be sterilized by autoclave, does not need cooling and can be stored at room temperature for about 2 years.

Further substances were suggested as foundations for viscoelastics but showed no clinical relevance (Karel et al., 1997).

CHAPTER 4

Product Specifications

Manufacturers' Information About Their Viscoelastics

In order to better interpret the information given by the manufacturer regarding viscosity, knowledge of the following relationships is crucial: the higher the molecular weight at low shear rates, the higher the viscosity (see above). Upon comparison of the information given by companies and manufacturers as to their viscoelastic products, the following discrepancies were noted: Morcher Oil® Plus is noted as having the same viscosity as Morcher Oil® in spite of both higher concentration and molecular weight; Healon® GV is listed as having 4 times higher viscosity at rest than Viscorneal® Plus, in spite of the same concentration and molecular weight (Fig. 29). Furthermore, companies producing viscoelastics for the same manufacturer (Bohus Biotech, Strömstad) list different information about the same viscoelastics agents (HSO® , Morcher Oil®, Microvisc®, HSO® Plus, Morcher Oil® Plus and Microvisc® Plus). These differences could be attributed to varying modes of calculation employed to derive zero shear viscosity, varying reference shear rates, different measuring instruments for rheologic examinations, perhaps even different environmental temperatures or batch dependent differences in molecular weight distribution.

Cool storage (2-8 °C) is generally required for both hyaluronate and hyaluronate-containing viscoelastics. They should be protected from long exposure to light and temperatures under 0 °C. Approximately 30 minutes prior to application, these preparations should be removed from their place of storage to attain room temperature for use. Cannula sizes of 25 (Rayvisc®), 27 (Healon®, Healon® GV, Provisc®, Viscoat®) and up to 30 G are recommended for injection of these viscoelastics.

Similar inconsistencies are seen in critical analyses of the information given for HPMC products (Fig. 30). Visco Shield®, for example, is listed as having a far higher molecular weight and supposedly a distinctly lower viscosity at rest than HPMC Ophtal® H, although their concentrations are cited as being the same. These variations prove that manufacturer information should be critically studied.

HPMC products can be stored at room temperature. Recommended cannula sizes for injection are between 20 G (Ocucoat®) and 25 G (HPMC Ophtal® L), i.e., wider cannula openings, as the pseudoplastic character of these viscoelastics is far less highlighted than in hyaluronic acid viscoelastics (see above).

product	polymer	concentration (%)	molecular weight (D)	viscosity (mPas)
Microvisc Plus	HA	1.4	7.9 Mio	n.i.
Morcher Oil Plus	HA	1.4	7.9 Mio	1 Mio
Morcher Oil	HA	1	6.1 Mio	1 Mio
Microvisc	HA	1	5 Mio	n.i.
Healon GV	HA	1.4	5 Mio	2 Mio
Viscorneal Plus	HA	1.4	5 Mio	500 000
Allervisc Plus	HA	1.4	5 Mio	500 000
Viscorneal	HA	1	5 Mio	200 000
Allervisc	HA	1	5 Mio	200 000
Healon5	HA	2.3	4 Mio	7 Mio
HSO Plus	HA	1.4	4 Mio	4.8 Mio
HSO	HA	1	4 Mio	1 Mio
Healon	HA	1	4 Mio	200 000
Dispasan Plus	HA	1.5	>3 Mio	2.5 Mio
Visko Plus	HA	1.4	3 Mio	500 000
BioLon	HA	1	3 Mio	115 000
Dispasan	HA	1	>2 Mio	35 000
Visko	HA	1	2 Mio	300 000
HYA-Ophtal	HA	2	2 Mio	n.i.
Amvisc Plus	HA	1.6	1.5 Mio	60 000
IALUM	HA	1.2	1.2 Mio	10 000
IALUM-F	HA	1.8	1.2 Mio	22 000
Provisc	HA	1	>1.1 Mio	50 000
Rayvisc	HA	3	800 000	50 000
AMO Vitrax	HA	3	500 000	40 000
Viscoat	HA	3	>500 000	ca. 40 000
	CS	4	22 500	

Fig. 29. Comparative listing of the properties (concentration, molecular weight, and viscosity at a shear rate of 0) of a selection of various commercially available hyaluronic-acid-based products (listed by declining molecular weight values; as described by the manufacturer); n.i. = no information provided

Our Own Comparative Trials

Motivated by the above related circumstances, we set out to compare all currently available viscoelastics on the German market using Advanced Rheometric Expansion System (Fig. 31; ARES) and RMS 800 (Rheometric Scientific Inc., Piscataway, USA) as our measuring systems with regard to their physicochemical pro-

product	polymer	concentration %	molecular weight (D)	viscosity (mPas)
LA GEL	HPMC	1.8	1.3 Mio	40 000
Visco Shield 2 %	HPMC	2	800 000	40 000
HPMC-Ophtal H	HPMC	2	250 000	55 000
Acrivisc	HPMC	2	86 000	4 500
Adatocel	HPMC	2	86 000	4 500
PeHa-Visco	HPMC	2	85 000	4 500
Celoftal	HPMC	2	80 000	4 000
Ocucoat	HPMC	2	80 000	4 000
HPMC-Ophtal L	HPMC	2	80 000	4 800
Coatel	HPMC	2	> 8 500	5 000

Fig. 30. Comparative listing of the properties (concentration, molecular weight, and viscosity at a shear rate of 0) of a selection of various commercially available hydroxypropylmethylcellulose-products (listed by declining molecular weight as described by the manufacturer)

perties. To describe the viscoelastic characteristics of a substance, 3 parameters are generally used: the elasticity modulus (G'), the viscosity modulus (G") and the phase angle (d). A rheometer calculates the complex modulus (G*) and the phase angle, out of which the elasticity and viscosity moduli are calculated.

The shear moduli, G', the elasticity modulus and G", the viscosity modulus, were determined. The elasticity modulus is defined as the relationship of elastic pressure (in phase) to the applied force and is dependent on the ability of a substance to store energy elastically. It represents a measure of the number of interactions in a specific system. The value of the elasticity modulus G' is proportional to the

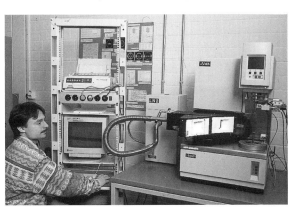

Fig. 31. The ARES rheometer was used for rheological investigations (geometry of the measuring device: conusplate; diameter: d=25 mm; angle: α=0.1 rad)

number of interactions and the strength of each interaction. The viscosity modulus G" describes the viscous part of a viscoelastic system; the higher the viscosity, the higher the value of the viscosity modulus.

$$G' = G^* \times \cos \delta \, (\tau'/\gamma) = \text{elasticity module}$$
$$G'' = G^* \times \sin \delta \, (\tau''/\gamma) = \text{viscosity module}$$

The phase angle (δ) describes the phase shift between the τ-vectors and is a measure of the degree of viscosity of a substance. A completely viscous (Newtonian) substance shows a phase angle of 90°, while a completely elastic (Hookian) body shows a phase angle of 0°. Interwoven polymer networks show a phase angle between 0° and 90°. Generally, the following relationship applies:

$$\tan \delta = G'' / G'$$
$$\tau' = \text{stress} = \text{stress constant} \times \text{torque (g} \times \text{cm)}$$
$$\gamma = \text{strain} = \text{strain constant} \times \text{shearing angle of motor (radians)}$$

The viscosity is a function of the applied stress and is named dynamic viscosity η' and complex viscosity η^*:

$$\eta' = G'' / \omega$$
$$\eta^* = [(G')^2 + (G'')^2 \, / \, \omega \,]^{-2}$$

where ω represents the frequency covered by the circle and, thereby, corresponds to the frequency multiplied by 2π.

As to the prevailing measurement conditions, the following becomes obvious: room temperature was 23°C, duration of measure in ARES totaled 10 minutes per preparation, not exceeded in any measurement. Measurements were taken beginning at the high frequencies, down to the low frequencies.

The test for dynamic frequency-dependency of complex viscosity η^* was used as the measuring method for each substance. Relaxation time was calculated from G' to G" above the intersection point, and the zero shear viscosity was mathematically derived by means of the so-called Ellis-fit (Fig. 32). The viscosity model, according to Ellis allows the calculation of zero shear viscosity using the following formula (compare Fig. 32):

$$y = \frac{c_1}{[1 + \frac{x}{c_2}]^{c_3 - 1}}$$

Zero shear viscosity η_0 represents a function of c_1. The following Figure 32 relates the Ellis model coefficient to the viscoelastic data.

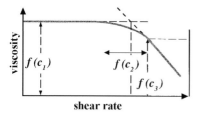

Fig. 32. Mathematical extrapolation of the zero shear viscosity using the Ellis-fit method: The viscosity is a function of c_1. The transitional stage between the amplitude of viscosity and the straight line (extrapolated) is a function of c_2. The first point of the diagonally directed straight line showing a constant ascend (law of power) will be described as function of c_3

Furthermore, pH-values were measured by a pH-meter (type CG 818, Schott Equipment, Hofheim, Germany). The measurements were taken from a total of 6 different viscoelastic vials per product, which were supplied, mostly free of charge, by the participating companies for the purpose of this trial.

The duration of measurements and the influence exerted by prolonged measuring time on rheologic viscoelastic results was examined within the context of pilot studies. Both the examined hyaluronic acid products as well as the HPMC products evaluated, showed a substantial reduction of viscoelastic mass after a maximum of 15 minutes (Fig. 33, 34). This relationship had never before been described in the literature. With prolonged measuring times, viscosity values were

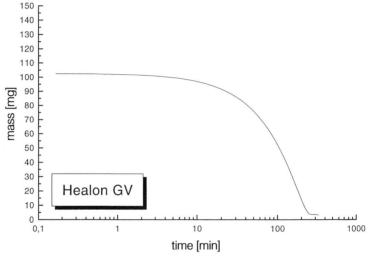

Fig. 33. Decreasing weight of a hyaluronic-acid-based product (Healon® GV) with increasing time

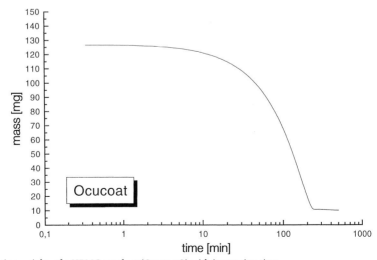

Fig. 34. Decreasing weight of a HPMC-product (Ocucoat®) with increasing time

considerably higher due to mass reduction, most likely a result of evaporation of viscoelastic water content (Fig. 35). Ten minutes were, therefore, established as an adequate interval for each measurement.

To relate the practical relevance of these results, specific requirement profiles for individual procedures have been correlated to the desired physicochemical characteristics (Table 5). Then, the viscoelastic which best fulfills these requirements (Arshinoff, 1991) is shown based on our own results.

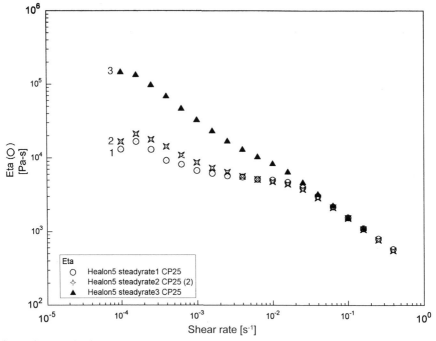

Fig. 35. The example of Healon®5 clearly shows that viscosity (especially with shear rates in low ranges) will increase when the time of measurement is increased (steadyrate 1-3; fixed points of time when measurements took place: 1=immediate start of measurements after loading the cell; 2=15 minutes after loading the cell; 3=30 minutes after loading the cell). This diagram shows how important it is to limit the time period of the measuring process

Table 5. Important characteristics of a viscoelastic substance during the various steps of catararact surgery (phacoemulsification/ECCE)

surgical step	shear rate (sec⁻¹)	characteristic
fill the anterior chamber	1 000-10 000	high pseudoplasticity
capsulorhexis/capsulotomy	0	high viscosity/elasticity
emulsification	-	low cohesion
expell the nucleus	2-5	pseudoplasticity
I/A cortex	-	coatability
fill the capsular bag	1 000	pseudoplasticity
keep the capsular bag open	0	high viscosity/elasticity
IOL implantation	5-10	pseudoplasticity
removal of the viscoelastic	-	cohesion

In cataract operations, high pseudoplasticity is desirable to inject the viscoelastic substance into the anterior chamber; capsulotomy and capsulorhexis require a high viscosity (Arshinoff, 1992), and nuclear extraction with ECCE necessitates pseudoplasticity. For phacoemulsification, low cohesive viscoelastic properties should be sought so that the viscoelastic does not leave the eye as a whole following the insertion of the phacoemulsification tip. During irrigation/aspiration of the cortex, good wetting and coating ability is desirable. For quick and easy filling of the capsular bag, high pseudoplasticity is required, where as keeping the capsular bag open demands high viscosity at low shear rate. During IOL implantation, increasing shear rates of 5-10 per second occur, necessitating high pseudoplasticity to avoid resistance during the operation (Arshinoff, 1986). For the implantation of foldable lenses, high elastic viscoelastics are beneficial, giving way to the lens during unfolding and again resuming their original form once the lens is in place. High cohesiveness allows for facilitated removal of viscoelastic, e.g,. in bolus form.

Zero Shear Viscosity

Of the currently internationally available hyaluronic acid-containing viscoelastic preparations, Healon®5, Healon® GV and Microvisc® Plus have the highest viscosity at rest, followed by Viscorneal® Plus (also sold by Allergan, Ettlingen, Germany, by the name Allervisc®, previously Ivisc® Plus), and Microvisc® (also sold by Morcher, Stuttgart, Germany, as Morcher Oil® (Plus) or by Polytech, Roßdorf, Germany, by the name HSO®) (Table 6; compare Figure 29, Manufacturers). Following, in decreasing order, are: Dispasan® (also Ophthalin®) Plus, Allervisc® (Viscorneal®), BioLon Prime™, Healon®, BioLon™ and Provisc® with medium viscosity at rest. Biocorneal®, Amvisc® Plus, Amvisc®, HYA-Ophtal®, Viscoat® and AMO Vitrax® belong to the group of hyaluronic acid-containing viscoelastics with the lowest zero shear viscosity values.

With HPMC products, viscosity at rest was hardly demonstrable, as expected. The exception was made by HPMC Ophtal® H and LA GEL® which showed higher viscosity, such as seen in some hyaluronic acid products. In contrast, Adatocel® Acrivisc® HPMC Ophtal L® Coatel® PeHa-Visco® and Ocucoat® all showed rather low zero shear viscosity values (Fig. 36, Table 6).

The viscoelastic behavioral profile of HPMC Ophthal® H corresponded closely with Amvisc® Plus, a hyaluronic acid product. Compared to the remaining HPMC products, a slight pseudoplastic property was recognized in this product, similar to hyaluronic acid products. These results support the conclusion that categorizing viscoelastics in substance groups does not always make evident their functional differences.

Pseudoplasticity

High shear rates are usually reached during injection of viscoelastics. The initial resistance is therefore perceptibly high, due to the high zero shear viscosity. Once the plunger starts to move, the viscosity of the substance decreases due to the higher shear rates, allowing the viscoelastic to be injected with little energy expenditure.

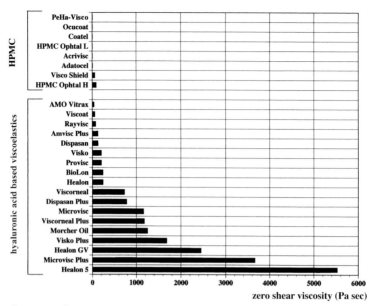

Fig. 36. Zero shear viscosity η_0 (sorted according to classes of substances in rising order; n=6)

Table 6. Zero shear viscosity [Pa sec; after extrapolation using the Ellis-fit; mean value (n = 6)]

product	zero shear viscosity (Pas)
Acrivisc®	7.3
Adatocel®	8.3
AMO Vitrax®	41.3
Amvisc®	106.5
Amvisc Plus®	128.2
Biocorneal®	166.2
BioLon™	243.2
BioLon Prime™	502.8
Coatel®	6.4
Dispasan® (Ophthalin®)	130.7
Dispasan Plus®	782.4
Healon®	243.3
Healon® GV	2 451.4
Healon®5	5 524.6
HPMC Ophtal® H	93.7
HPMC Ophtal® L	7.0
HYA-Ophtal®	78.5
LA GEL®	53.8
Microvisc® (HSO)®	1 162.6
Microvisc® (HSO)® Plus	3 662.7
Morcher Oil® GV	1 253.3
Ocucoat®	5.9
PeHa-Visco®	5.0
Provisc®	207.3
Rayvisc®	77.5
Viscoat®	58.3
Viscorneal® (Allervisc®)	732.9
Viscorneal® (Allervisc®) Plus	1 176.0
Visco Shield®	59.7
Visko® 1 %	205.9
Visko® 1.4 %	1 682.9

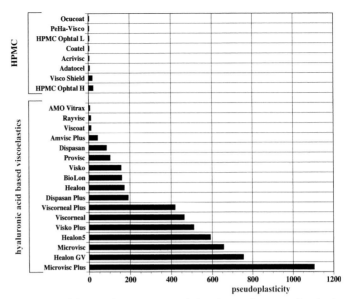

Fig. 37. Pseudoplasticity P_2 (quotient of the zero shear viscosity and viscosity at a shear rate of 100/sec); sorted according to classes of substances and range of pseudoplasticity, in rising order; n=6)

Table 7. Pseudoplasticity P_1 (quotient of the viscosity at a shear rate of 0.1/sec and the viscosity at 100/sec) and pseudoplasticity P_2 [quotient of the zero shear viscosity extrapolated using the Ellis-fit and the viscosity at a shear rate of 100/sec); mean value (n = 6)]

product	viscosity η (0.1/sec)	viscosity η (100/sec)	P_1	P_2
Acrivisc®	11.32	1.45	7.81	5.03
Adatocel®	3.76	1.39	2.70	5.97
AMO Vitrax®	39.21	6.18	6.34	6.68
Amvisc Plus®	120.89	2.99	40.43	42.88
BioLon™	175.18	1.52	115.25	160.00
Coatel®	5.48	1.41	3.90	4.53
Dispasan® (Ophthalin®)	66.66	1.52	43.86	85.99
Dispasan Plus®	78.25	4.09	19.13	191.30
Healon®	156.76	1.41	111.18	172.55
Healon® GV	783.27	3.25	241.01	754.27
Healon®5	2357.22	9.34	252.46	591.50
HPMC Ophtal® H	78.25	4.09	19.13	22.91
HPMC Ophtal® L	6.67	1.52	4.39	4.61
HYA-Ophtal®	65.33	2.91	22.45	26.96
LA GEL®	40.25	2.51	16.04	21.41
Microvisc®	689.63	1.77	389.62	656.84
Microvisc® Plus	1824.3	3.32	549.49	1103.22
Morcher Oil®	723.02	1.91	378.54	656.15
Ocucoat®	7.71	1.61	4.79	3.67
PeHa-Visco®	5.74	1.23	4.65	4.07
Provisc®	140.45	2.00	70.23	103.65
Rayvisc®	74.41	7.04	10.58	11.01
Viscoat®	51.01	5.03	10.14	11.59
Viscorneal® (Allervisc®)	291.86	1.58	184.72	463.86
Viscorneal® (Allervisc®) Plus	536.73	2.80	191.69	420.00
Visco Shield®	43.08	3.11	13.86	19.20
Visko®	132.78	1.31	101.08	157.21
Visko® Plus	691.02	3.29	209.93	511.25

Two quotients, P_1 and P_2, were established as measures for pseudoplasticity (Fig. 37, Table 7).

Relaxation Time

When performing phacoemulsification under topical anesthesia, the outer eye muscles retain their tone explaining the absence of a "soft" eye and, for example, possibly a raised vitreous pressure. Raised vitreous pressure may encumber capsulorhexis or IOL implantation because of narrowed anterior chamber conditions (Fig. 38).

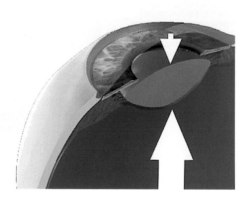

Fig. 38. An increased vitreal pressure calls for an antagonistic substance which under pressure will not immediately leave the eye through an opening. Thus the viscoelastic substance should feature a high viscosity at rest

Besides high substance viscosity at zero shear rate, constant space-occupying effectiveness is indispensable in such cases as some viscoelastics alter their molecular configuration when experiencing external pressure, even without application of shear force, and, thereby, also change their viscosity at rest. The so-called relaxation time reflects the duration of space-occupying effectiveness and is determined by the intersection of G'/G". HPMC products, such as Acrivisc®, Adatocel®, Coatel®, HPMC Ophtal® L, Ocucoat®, and PeHa-Visco®, show practically no space-occupying effectiveness while HPMC Ophtal® H and Visco Shield® show space-occupying effectiveness of very short duration (Fig. 39, Table 8). This suggests that no HPMC product fulfills the rheologic criteria demanded of a viscoelastic for cataract operations with high vitreous pressure. Although the hyaluronic acid products AMO Vitrax®, Amvisc®, Amvisc® Plus, Biocorneal®, Dispasan®, HYA-Ophtal®, Provisc®, Rayvisc®, Viscoat®, Viscorneal®, and Viscorneal® only showed space-occupying effectiveness for a short duration; most were effective longer than the HPMC products. BioLon™, BioLon Prime™, Dispasan® Plus, Healon®, Visco®, Visco® Plus, and especially Healon® GV, Healon®5, Microvisc® (HSO® Morcher Oil®), and Microvisc® Plus have shown space-occupying effectiveness for longer durations of time (Fig. 39).

Relaxation behavior of a high viscous and a low viscous viscoelastic was measured and is represented in Figures 40 and 41.

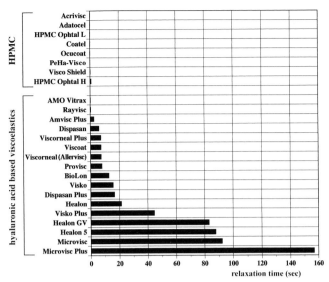

Fig. 39. Mean relaxation time (sec) as a value for the period of the space tactical effectivity of a visco-elastic substance (sorted according to the classes of substances and the period of the relaxation time, both with rising order; n=6)

Table 8. Mean relaxation time (sec) as a measure for duration of the space tactical effectivity of a visco-elastic substance (n = 6)

product	relaxation time (sec)
Acrivisc®	0.06
Adatocel®	0.06
AMO Vitrax®	0.17
Amvisc®	2.57
Amvisc Plus®	2.50
Biocorneal®	5.50
BioLon™	12.65
BioLon Prime™	15.14
Coatel®	0.06
Dispasan® (Ophthalin®)	5.99
Dispasan Plus®	16.57
Healon®	21.40
Healon® GV	83.19
Healon®5	87.91
HPMC Ophtal® H	0.75
HPMC Ophtal® L	0.06
HYA-Ophtal®	0.99
LA GEL®	0.25
Microvisc® (HSO)®	92.40
Microvisc® (HSO)® Plus	156.89
Morcher Oil®	90.76
Ocucoat®	0.06
PeHa-Visco®	0.06
Provisc®	7.93
Rayvisc®	0.32
Viscoat®	7.32
Viscorneal® (Allervisc®)	7.44
Viscorneal® (Allervisc®) Plus	7.30
Visco Shield®	0.20
Visko®	15.62
Visko® Plus	44.65

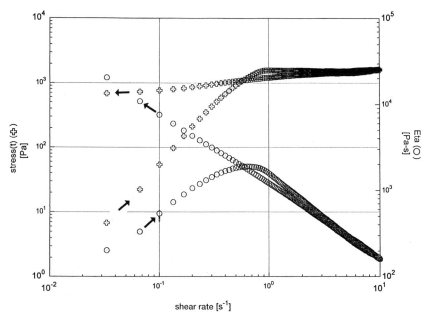

Fig. 40. After the excitation of a highly viscous viscoelastic substance (Healon® GV, arrow pointing right) Healon® GV will keep its new shape (in ranges of high viscosity) for a relatively long period of time even under pressure (arrow pointing now to the left). Thus the resulting relaxation time (sec) is also prolonged (compare with Table 8)

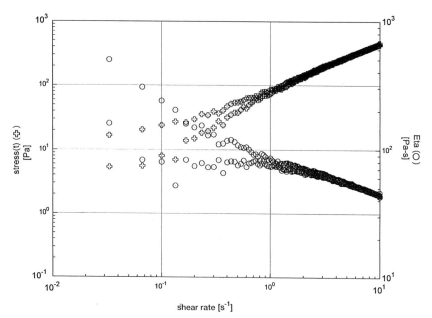

Fig. 41. After the excitation of a low-viscous viscoelastic substance (Ocucoat®, for explanation see above) the new shape (in ranges of low viscosity, right y-axis) will hardly be kept under exceeding pressure. Thus the resulting relaxation time (sec) is also short

Intersection G' / G" (Elasticity modulus / viscosity modulus)

When implanting foldable intraocular lenses, a deep, stable anterior chamber is as crucial as even posterior capsule extension. When using injectors, viscoelastics can serve as coating (see below). The viscoelastic should be easily removed following implantation, which is more easily achieved with cohesive viscoelastics. In summary, high viscosity and relatively high elasticity at low shear rates would be ideal. These characteristics are particularly well seen in the following viscoelastic substances: Healon®5, followed by Healon® GV, Microvisc® Plus, and Viscorneal®/Allervisc® (Table 9, Fig. 42). Viscoelastic substances whose G'/G" intersection lies to the left of frequency 1 feel elastic to the touch, while viscoelastic substances whose G'/G" intersection lies to the right of 1 feel viscous to the touch (Fig. 42). For the implantation of foldable intraocular lenses, high viscosity and elasticity at medium shear rates (0.1 rad/sec) is desirable. Viscoelastics to the right of 1 with a high G'/G" intersection are especially suitable (Fig. 42, also compare Fig. 43 and 44).

Table 9. Alphabetical listing of the viscoelastic substances with their G'/G" cross point and frequency (rad/sec and 1/sec)

product	G'/G" intersection (Pa)	frequency (rad/sec)	frequency (Hz)
Acrivisc®	–	>100	15.916
Adatocel®	–	>100	15.917
AMO Vitrax®	287.70	37.812	6.018
Amvisc Plus®	64.90	2.522	0.401
BioLon™	25.40	0.497	0.079
Coatel®	–	>100	15.914
Dispasan®	26.69	1.048	0.167
Dispasan Plus®	60.98	0.379	0.060
Healon®	19.36	0.294	0.047
Healon® GV	53.24	0.076	0.0120
Healon®5	142.38	0.072	0.0115
HPMC Ophtal® H	109.57	8.433	1.342
HPMC Ophtal® L	–	>100	15.915
HYA-Ophtal®	79.86	6.330	1.007
LA GEL®	93.30	24.980	3.975
Microvisc® (HSO®)	24.46	0.068	0.011
Microvisc® (HSO®) Plus	51.49	0.040	0.006
Morcher Oil®	26.28	0.069	0.011
Ocucoat®	–	>100	15.916
PeHa-Visco®	–	>100	15.918
Provisc®	34.62	0.793	0.126
Rayvisc®	268.87	19.665	3.130
Viscoat®	175.26	16.20	2.579
Viscorneal® (Allervisc®)	22.15	0.125	0.020
Viscorneal® (Allervisc®) Plus	45.94	0.157	0.025
Visco Shield®	132.92	31.129	4.954
Visko®	20.61	0.402	0.064
Visko® Plus	65.77	0.141	0.022

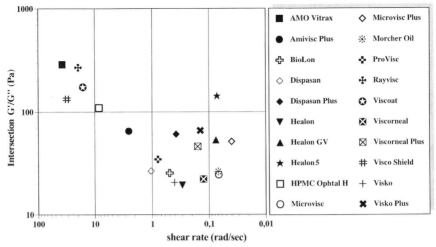

Fig. 42. The G'/G" (Pa) cross point serves as a characteristic to describe the extent of viscosity and elasticity of a viscoelastic substance and their according frequencies (in alphabetical order; n=6). The elastical properties of a viscoelastic substance will dominate with increasing frequencies (to a different extent; compare with the individual graphs). Due to the division by 2π the unit rad/sec wil be exchanged into Hertz (Hz). In the case of 5 HPMC-products no cross point could be determined for they should exceed (have to be located outside of) the 100 rad/sec value. The rheological characteristics mentioned above are better described by the following example (Figure 43 and 44)

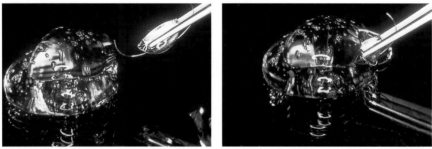

Fig. 43-44. A foldable IOL is introduced into a high viscous hyaluronic acid viscoelastic substance (Healon®5) without harming the outer shape of the viscoelastic substance significantly. Despite its high viscosity at rest the product obviously shows a high pseudoplasticity and elasticity (compare with table 7)

pH-Value

The pH of aqueous humor is normally 7.38. Undamaged human endothelium can largely compensate for the damaging effects of intraocularly applied solutions within a pH range between 6.8 and 8.1. Beyond this range, irreversible corneal ultrastructural and functional alterations occur (Gonnering et al., 1979). Compromised endothelium, such as cornea guttata or Fuchs endothelial dystrophy, demonstrate substantially lower pH-values. Four viscoelastic substances have average pH-values clearly outside the aforementioned range (Fig. 45, Table 10). Brief contact between these solutions with pH-value 6.5 and human endothelial cells will lead to swelling of the cells and their organelles, as well as widening of the intercellular spaces (Fig. 46 and 47).

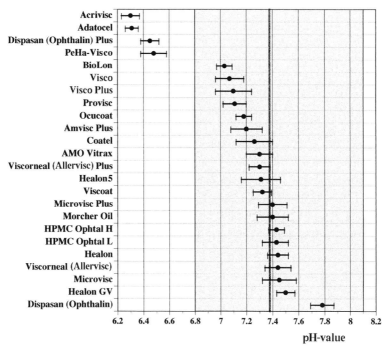

Fig. 45. Mean pH-values of different viscoelastic substances when taking in account the pH-value of the anterior chamber of the eye (7.38) as well as the compensational pH-value range from 6.6 to 8.1 (sorted according to increasing pH-values; n=6)

Table 10. Mean pH-values of various viscoelastic substances (6 different vials)

product	pH-value (mean ± SD)
Acrivisc®	6.3 (±0.07)
Adatocel®	6.31 (±0.05)
Dispasan (Ophthalin®) Plus®	6.45 (±0.07)
PeHa-Visco®	6.48 (±0.1)
BioLon™	7.03 (±0.06)
Visko®	7.07 (±0.11)
Visko® Plus	7.1 (±0.14)
Provisc®	7.11 (±0.09)
Ocucoat®	7.18 (±0.06)
Amvisc Plus®	7.2 (±0.12)
Coatel®	7.26 (±0.14)
AMO Vitrax®	7.3 (±0.10)
Viscorneal® (Allervisc®) Plus	7.3 (±0.08)
Healon®5	7.31 (±0.15)
Viscoat®	7.32 (±0.07)
Microvisc® (HSO)® Plus	7.4 (±0.11)
Morcher Oil®	7.4 (±0.12)
HPMC Ophtal® H	7.43 (±0.06)
HPMC Ophtal® L	7.43 (±0.09)
Healon®	7.44 (±0.08)
Viscorneal® (Allervisc®)	7.44 (±0.10)
Microvisc® (HSO)®	7.45 (±0.13)
Healon® GV	7.5 (±0.07)
Dispasan® (Ophthalin®)	7.78 (±0.09)

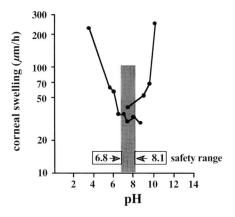

Fig. 46. Influence of the pH-value of a solution on corneal swelling: In the pH-value range from 6.8 to 8.1 only a small swelling of the cornea takes place (logarithmic presentation modified according to Gonnering et al., 1979)

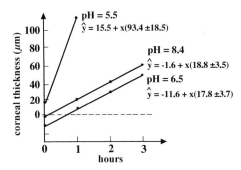

Fig. 47. The thickness of the human cornea changes dependent on the pH-value of the solution (modified according to Gonnering et al., 1979)

CHAPTER 5

General Applications of Viscoelastics

The many and diverse physicochemical characteristics of viscoelastic substances impose both their desired and undesired effects clinically. As there is no single ideal substance to meet clinical stipulations, individual viscoelastic characteristics should be considered with respect to demand. Georg Eisner described viscoelastic agents as a tool for space-occupying measures (in tissues, in space or on surfaces) applied by the use of special techniques (Eisner, 1980; Eisner, 1983). In surgery, viscoelastic substances protect tissues and cells from mechanical trauma, serve to separate tissues, occupy space, break away adhesions, stop bleeding, coat, act as manipulative instruments and move tissues back and forth. Furthermore, they maintain space postoperatively for a certain amount of time and can reduce local bleeding. Side-effects are noted as well. As opposed to pure fluids, viscoelastic substances do not spread out throughout the entire intraocular space, but rather remain mostly around the area of injection. Since viscoelastic substances consume space, it follows that they require adequate space or compressible tissue might be displaced. Possible consequences include, for example, further radial tearing and rupture of the posterior lens capsule, lesions in the zonula or iris and lastly, lens or implant luxation.

Viscoelastic substances are occasionally difficult to remove. In general, Viscoat® and HPMC products are more difficult to aspirate than sodium hyaluronate. Viscoelastic residues leave the eye by means of the trabecular meshwork and drainage canals, resulting in increased intraocular pressure, particularly in the presence of other risk factors (e.g., glaucoma) which encumber drainage. Although sodium hyaluronate is removed from the aqueous humor of monkey eyes within 72 hours, the half-life of sodium hyaluronate, following injection into the vitreous body of the owl-monkey eye, is 72 days. It is also conceivable that the eye further processes metabolic by-products of, for example, HPMC. Viscoelastic substances absorb blood and fibrin which can bring about inflammation once the viscoelastic is transported beyond the area of injection.

As a rule, reuse of remaining viscoelastic substance or splitting up a unit for application in more than one operation should be avoided.

Maintenance of the Anterior Chamber

Viscosity and elasticity are the general rheologic characteristics influencing the maintenance of the anterior chamber. Theoretically, the higher the viscosity, the better the maintenance of chamber depth at rest; i.e., at zero shear rate. Based on an in-vitro study performed by Miyauchi and Iwata (1986) involving a model with different viscosity and elasticity, it was shown that the ability to maintain space in the anterior chamber is far more dependent upon the elasticity than the viscosity.

HPMC products are not suitable to maintain anterior chamber depth with concomitant increased vitreous pressure due to their low elasticity. Higher molecular weight sodium hyaluronate was proven to be superior for this clinical application (Strobel, 1997).

In the case of intraoperative soft eye, almost all viscoelastic substances would be adequate. In clinical application, all currently available viscoelastic substances are capable of maintaining chamber depth, to some extent, without much difficulty (Liesegang, 1990).

Injection techniques, in the context of small-incision surgery, would depend upon whether the anterior chamber is deep or collapsed. A very shallow or collapsed anterior chamber will seldom occur intraoperatively (e.g., during complicated cataract surgery) or postoperatively (e.g., following complicated cataract surgery, fistulating glaucoma surgery or combined surgery). Fisher and co-workers (1982) first reported successful anterior chamber deepening with the use of hyaluronic acid, of a persistently flat anterior chamber following ICCE. In pseudophakia, anterior IOL displacement due to a flattened anterior chamber, can promote the development of peripheral anterior and posterior synechiae or, for instance, unwanted endothelial contact-damage. Iris-capture syndrome with pupillary block or angle closure represents other possible unwanted effects. The injection of a viscoelastic offers some advantages in this context:

- A temporarily deepened anterior chamber with mechanical separation of tissue compartments, which counteracts synechial formation as well as IOL contact with the corneal endothelium.
- Hindering drainage and permitting wound healing when the incision leaks
- Patients experience less discomfort associated with ocular hypotony and the collapse of the anterior chamber together with quickly improved vision.

Osher and co-workers (1996) described the deepening of the anterior chamber with Healon® following cataract operation and showed that it be sufficient to fill the anterior chamber halfway, instead of completely. However, it was pointed out that precaution be taken to carefully monitor IOP values to avoid potentially excessive rises.

Injection Techniques into a Deep Anterior Chamber

Viscoelastic is either injected within a safe distance of the access port or the drainage port, i.e., opposite or next to the incision, to allow unhindered aqueous drain-

Fig. 48. Technique to inject a viscoelastic substance in case of a deep anterior chamber

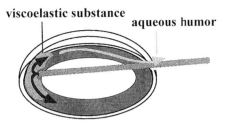

Fig. 48. Technique to inject a viscoelastic substance in case of a deep anterior chamber

age (Fig. 48). The tip of the injection cannula is dipped into the viscoelastic, particularly when using high viscous viscoelastic substances (those with high refractive indices) in order to inject a continuous stream and avoid any eventual diffraction zones which might obscure visibility. As the injection procedure continues, the cannula is moved towards the other opening without blocking it with viscoelastic. Should viscoelastic obscure the opening, compensatory aqueous drainage might become blocked and the intraocular pressure might rise, making difficult further injection of viscoelastic into the anterior chamber.

Injection Technique into a Collapsed Anterior Chamber

In contrast to the above technique, OVD injection begins during introduction of the cannula into the access port on its way into the intraocular space (Fig. 49) in order to move the iris towards the lens.

Further deposits are then applied along the circumference of the iris so as to displace the entire access to the area behind the iris. An inverted pupillary block is achieved, to an extent, which then allows the anterior chamber to deepen at the expense of the posterior chamber. Only now is the remaining anterior chamber space filled with viscoelastic.

ATTENTION: OVD injection opposite to the opening will push the iris either up or down peripherally. If it remains behind the iris, viscoelastic might press the iris upwards towards the access port (Fig. 50). Furthermore, viscoelastic in the retroiridal space is cumbersome to remove.

Fig. 49. The process of injecting a viscoelastic substance in case of a collapsed anterior chamber

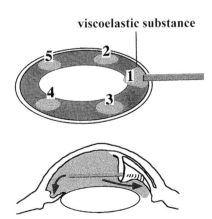

Fig. 50. Wrong technique to inject a viscoelastic substance in case of a collapsed anterior chamber

Tissue Manipulation

In anterior chamber surgery, viscoelastic substances are useful in displacing tissues, i.e., pushing tissue back out of the anterior chamber. They also help in extending the capsule to avoid it from curling up, allow capsulorhexis and separate tissue parts from one another. These applications are similar to those of maintaining anterior chamber space and require a viscoelastic substance with high viscosity, elasticity and pseudoplasticity. At rest or with slow movement within the anterior chamber, a high viscosity viscoelastic should be chosen to keep tissues apart. At a high shear rate within the cannula, corresponding to almost 10,000 per second during injection, the pseudoplasticity curves of currently available viscoelastic substances are comparable.

Viscomydriasis

Well aimed viscoelastic injections are helpful in widening the pupil. Injections should be aimed at the slightly raised portion of the iris (i.e., iris frill) and less at the pupil rim to prevent viscoelastic from getting behind the iris (Fig. 51). Since viscoelastic usually flows in all directions, a large amount will possibly be needed, depending on the depth of the anterior chamber. An injection of air directly beneath the cornea can help reduce the amount of viscoelastic required, with the possible disadvantage of poorer visibility into the eye, due to refractive irregularities.

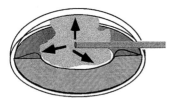

Fig. 51. Injection technique to create a mydriasis with the help of a viscoelastic substance

Facilitating Lens Implantation

In lens implantation, a viscoelastic substance is capable of giving more resistance than air or BSS (balanced salt solution). Furthermore, a viscoelastic offers other helpful properties, such as occupying and maintaining space and protecting the corneal endothelium. In the implantation of foldable lenses, the following rheologic characteristics are worth observing:

High viscous viscoelastic substances exert a compressive force through vertical pressure against the corneal endothelium. The movement of the IOL exerts drag and shear forces on the corneal endothelium, caused by the viscoelastic. Drag forces are slight with low viscous viscoelastics. Both forces can be transferred onto the endothelium through the viscoelastic in the anterior chamber and constitute sources of potential damage (see below).

Coatability

Both a high surface tension and a large contact angle contribute to poor wetting and coating ability. Viscoat® and HPMC show a lower surface tension and a smaller contact angle than sodium hyaluronate according to the literature. Clinically, this capacity allows viscoelastic substances to coat instruments and implants for longer. The surface tension was measured for comparison by Silver and co-workers (1994) with the following results: Healon® 62.7 ± 6.51 dynes/cm; Ocucoat® 43.0 ± 1.41 dynes/cm. Both low and high molecular weight HPMC show a lower surface tension than any hyaluronic acid preparations. This lower surface tension correlates with the formation of a coating layer on the endothelial surface. Generally, fluids disperse more when the surface tension of the fluid is lower than the critical surface tension of the tissue (Rodriguez, 1982). The critical surface tension of the corneal endothelium is between 43 and 63 dynes/cm, according to calculations made by Silver and co-workers (1994).

A common accompanying effect of a viscous, and therefore easily aspirated, viscoelastic is its poor coatability (e.g., sodium hyaluronate). It is possible that a microscopically thin layer of viscoelastic remains on the corneal endothelium following aspiration from the anterior chamber. Whether an increased coating ability has a protective influence on the corneal endothelium or not, is debated. It is conceivable that physically induced injury to the corneal endothelium may be indirectly caused by endothelial coating, due to drag forces exerted during aspiration of viscoelastic. Chemically induced injury to the endothelium may occur sooner if coatability is high.

The coating of the corneal epithelial surface, by contrast, causes moisture to be held in, keeping it smoother for a longer period of time and fostering good visibility. Frequent surface coating thus becomes unnecessary. The use of a large 'blob' can have similar effects to a Köppe-lens, permitting chamber angle visualization.

Corneal Endothelial Protection

Following damage, corneal epithelial cells can regenerate. A thick protective layer of glycoprotein from mucous secretions protects the epithelium from mechanical trauma. Endothelial cells, however, do not have the same potential to regenerate (e.g., mitosis).

Intraoperative factors as potential sources of injury to corneal endothelial cells are:
• Instruments
• Lens fragments
• IOL contact with the endothelium (Kassar &Varnell, 1982)
• Turbulence and volume of irrigation fluid (Edelhauser & MacRae, 1985; Glasser et al., 1985)
• Endothelial air bubbles (Craig et al., 1990)
• Free radicals from phacoemulsification (Holst et al., 1993)
• Sound wave conduction (Frohn et al., 1998), phacoemulsification performance and duration (Dick et al., 1996)

During operations, viscoelastic agents act as a sort of physical shield. Many physical properties contribute to endothelial protection:

- Occupying and maintaining space for intraocular manipulation
- Coating of endothelium and implant to avoid direct contact with instruments or IOL[1]
- Endothelial protection from shear- and compression forces
- Separation of tissue and implant on the one side, and endothelium on the other

The existence of specific sodium hyaluronate binding sites on the corneal endothelium has been established (Forsberg et al., 1994; Madsen et al., 1989a and 1989b; Härfstrand et al., 1992). This fact supports the suspicion that sodium hyaluronate might act as a natural endothelial shield during surgery (Stenevi et al., 1993). With regard to phacoemulsification, a protective corneal endothelial effect, by way of endothelial sodium hyaluronate receptor sites, is questionable. After phacoemulsification with IOL implantation in eyes with cornea guttata, Schmidl and co-workers (1998) found in an intraindividual trial conducted comparing 2 viscoelastic substances with different viscosity and molecular weight a statistically significant lower increase in corneal thickness in eyes having received the high viscosity viscoelastic (Healon® GV), compared to that observed in the other eye, managed with a low molecular weight viscoelastic with low viscosity. The lesser impairment of corneal endothelial function (by the higher molecular weight viscoelastic) could be attributed to the stronger affinity of endothelial hyaluronic acid receptor sites to high molecular weight hyaluronic acid.

Also, compression forces effect the corneal endothelium for instance, resulting from the direct conduction of pressure and sound waves across the viscoelastic (Hammer & Burch, 1984). High elastic viscoelastic substances conduct less compression force thereby lending better protection to the endothelium than air or BSS (Guthoff et al., 1992). Through movement and manipulation within the viscoelastic, parallel to the corneal surface, shear and drag forces can cause corneal endothelial damage, especially when using solutions of higher viscosity, higher elasticity or higher cohesiveness. When using BSS or air, damage due to conduction can be considered negligible (Arshinoff, 1989).

To provide the corneal endothelium with good protection, viscoelastic agents should ideally have high viscosity and elasticity at rest (zero shear rate). Such viscoelastic substances could protect the corneal endothelium from compression forces (Fig. 52). Additionally, the viscoelastic should have a steep pseudoplasticity curve, i.e., a quick viscosity reduction with increasing movement. Shear forces conducted to the corneal endothelium would, in this way, be minimized (Hammer & Burch, 1984).

As was seen in in-vitro and animal studies, 1% sodium hyaluronic acid, 10 & 20% chondroitin sulfate and 1% HPMC solutions protected the corneal endothelial cells from potential injury from direct contact of the IOL or instruments with corneal endothelium (Hammer & Burch, 1984; Miyauchi & Iwata, 1984). There is, however, no viscoelastic capable of shielding the corneal endothelium from sharp instruments, accentuating the importance of creating and maintaining a deep an-

---

[1] Keates, Powell & Blosser, 1987

Fig. 52. The force of compression acts vertically on the corneal endothelium and is lessened with the help of high-viscous viscoelastic substances. The movement of the IOL combined with the viscoelastic substance challenges the corneal endothelium due to drag and tractive forces. This shear force can be reduced by low viscous viscoelastic substances. Both forces will be influenced by the viscoelastic substance and are otherwise potentially harmful (modified according to Liesegang, 1990)

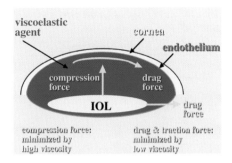

terior chamber as a means of corneal endothelial protection. Even a thin coat of medium or low viscous substance such as 0.17% sodium hyaluronate or 1% HPMC, will lend the endothelium a degree of protection by coating it (Hammer & Burch, 1984). A high viscous viscoelastic, such as hyaluronic acid, provides protection through the long-lasting maintenance of space when applied in a thick coat (rather than by coatability in a thin layer as seen above with high shear force conduction). This thick coating stops the implant from approaching the endothelium and counters the conduction of drag forces. Contact between the implant and the corneal endothelium could result in major endothelial damage with 1 % sodium hyaluronate solution through the conduction of drag forces. Frohn and co-workers (2000) examined sound wave conduction during phacoemulsification in a specially designed artificial eye, as related to different viscoelastic substances. As compared to BSS, sound waves were only slightly influenced by the HPMC medium (and sometimes increased) while all hyaluronic acid-containing preparations led to a reduction of sound amplitude arriving at the corneal endothelium complex and thereby, a reduction in sound conduction (Table 11). The clinical significance of sound wave conduction to the cornea is not clearly determined. However, there is evidence to support that high frequency ultrasound induce cell injury (Buschmann, 1997; Charliet & Crowet, 1986).

Chemical OVD properties play a large role in the complex interactions with the endothelium. Microscopic examinations (specular, scanning electron and transmission) of the cornea revealed that 1% sodium hyaluronate called forth no

Table 11. Sensor output (mean mV ± standard deviation) of the viscoelastic agents proportional to the amplitude. Ten measurements were made of all preparations

product	Sensor Output (Mean mV ± SD)
BSS	83.1 ± 6.21
Hydroxypropylmethylcellulose derivatives	
Adataocel®	97.9 ± 7.53
HPMC Ophtal H®	79.0 ± 4.01
Hyaluronic-acid-containing derivatives	
Healon®	74.1 ± 3.91
Viscorneal® Plus	68.5 ± 3.31
Healon® GV	65.1 ± 1.83
Provisc®	60.3 ± 9.75
Viscoat®	47.7 ± 2.50
Dispasan® Plus (Ophthalin®)	31.6 ± 4.12

Table 12. In-vitro studies on the protective effect of different viscoelastic substances on the corneal endothelium

author	year	cornea	method	results
Glasser	1986	rabbit	PMMA IOL abrasion test	ns: HY, HPMC, V
Glasser	1989	rabbit	phaco ± traumatic IOL implantation	without: ns with: V > HY
Condon	1989	human	cornea in viscoelastics	V, HPMC > HY
Craig	1990	human	phaco ± air bubble damage (Healon®: 4.9%; Viscoat®: 0.3%)	V > HY
Glasser	1991	rabbit	traumatic IOL implantation	V > HY
Monson	1991	human	phaco ± air bubble damage (Healon®: 4.3%; Ocucoat®: 1.4%)	HPMC > HY
Ngyuen	1992	bovine ECL	fluid model	HY > V
Artola	1993	rabbit	damage by free radicals (peroxidation)	HPMC > HY (for 1 & 10 mM) HY > HPMC (for 100 mM)
Bresciani	1996	pork	traumatic phaco (Healon®: 14.3%; Viscoat®: 2.5%)	V > HY
Poyer	1998	ECL	retention of viscoelastics following I/A	V > HY
McDermott	1998	rabbit	phaco via clear corneal tunnel; quantitative determination of the viscoelastic layer	V > HY

ECL = endothelial cell line, HY = hyaluronate-based viscoelastic substance, HPMC = hydroxypropyl-methylcellulose, V = Viscoat® (4% chondroitin sulfate and 3% hyaluronate), > = more than, ns = not statistically significant

toxic endothelial reaction (Graue, Polack & Balazs, 1980). Similarly, 1% sodium hyaluronic acid, 0.4% HPMC and 10% & 20% chondroitin sulfate exerted no adverse effects on the corneal endothelium (MacRae et al., 1983). Following human in-vitro corneal endothelial exposure to various viscoelastic agents for up to 20 minutes, significantly less cell toxicity (mitochondrial degeneration, intracellular vacuole degeneration) was observed in response to prolonged exposure to Healon® than HPMC or Viscoat® (Condon et al., 1989; table 12). The authors related these findings to the high viscosity with high shear force exertion, and the galenical constitution with a calcium-free vehicle. Chondroitin sulfate, Viscoat® and HPMC were less well tolerated with respect to certain cell parameters. In a similar trial, the cause of cell toxicity was associated with the osmolality of chondroitin sulfate (Meyer & McCulley, 1989). The high calcium-binding affinity of chondroitin sulfate could possibly contribute to the maintenance of (or even increase in) extracellular calcium levels. Critics have contended that the examination system devised does not reflect the actual, clinical conditions, as BSS-rinsing solutions were used, as well as calcium, which are not constituents of aqueous fluid. Many viscoelastic substances contain neither calcium nor magnesium, as these cations could evoke precipitation. Toxic effects on the corneal endothelium could also result from long-standing deficiency of these, which the application of chondroitin sulfate possibly avoids. Rinsing with 20% chondroitin sulfate substantially reduces corneal endothelial thickness associated with the substance's high osmolality and correlated dehydrating effects. During corneal transplantation this dehydration could be detrimental.

Endothelial protection provided by viscoelastics during primary and secondary lens implantation has been displayed in numerous clinical trials. Although air led to less endothelial cell damage than BSS (Bourne, Brubaker & O'Fallon, 1979), long-term exposure of the corneal endothelium to air proved toxic (Eiferman & Wilkins, 1981). Early tests showed less endothelial cell loss through the use of Healon®, in contrast to control groups (Miller & Stegmann, 1981; Pape, 1980a and 1980b).

It has been substantiated, without a doubt, that application of sodium hyaluronate during complicated surgical procedures shields the corneal endothelium (Balazs, 1986a; Miller & Stegmann, 1982; Rashid & Waring, 1982; Roper-Hall, 1983). Few trials resulted in as high an endothelium shielding capacity as air during uncomplicated extracapsular cataract extraction or phacoemulsification (Bourne et al., 1984; Hoffer, 1982).

The fact that the vast majority of authors found no significant differences regarding endothelial cell loss and corneal thickness following the use of viscoelastics in cataract surgery in comparable clinical trials comparing different viscoelastics is key (Table 13).

Table 13. Selection of comparative studies (inclusion criteria: prospective, randomized, number of eyes ≥ 40, endothelial cell analysis 4 weeks postoperatively at earliest, phacoemulsification in the capsular bag)

author, year	number	viscoelastic substance	endothelial cell loss	P	corneal thickness
Rafuse, 1992	60	HY/Viscoat®	2.7%/9.3%	ns	ns
Koch, 1993	59	HY/Viscoat®	0.6%/6.5% (central)	ns	ns
			9.9%/3.3% (superior)	ns	ns
Probst, 1993	50	HY/Viscoat®	11.1%/10.1%	ns	ns
Ravalico, 1997	66	HY/Healon® GV/ Viscoat®/HPMC	8.0%/7.6%/7.6%/8.8%	ns	ns

HY = hyaluronic acid based viscoelastic, HPMC = hydroxypropylmethylcellulose, ns = not statistically significant

Similarly, after use in ECCE, many clinical studies revealed insignificant or clinically irrelevant differences in endothelial cell loss and corneal thickness when comparing different viscoelastics. (Alpar, 1985; Alpar et al., 1988; Lane, 1991; Smith & Lindstrom, 1991). In a trial led by Pederson (1990), central corneal thickness was statistically significant higher following phacoemulsification and use of HPMC products than Healon®.

Hemostasis

The glycosaminoglycans, sodium hyaluronate and chondroitin sulfate, bear structural resemblance to heparin. Several studies have demonstrated a slight anticoagulative effect of these materials (Pandolfi & Hedner, 1984). Viscoelastic substances work hemostatically which is caused predominantly through tamponade (Packer et al., 1985).

Management of Complications

Next to proper technique, the suitable selection of a viscoelastic is vital in controlling complications.

Regarding OVD application with intraoperative complications, tissue stability and movement must be differentiated from selective tissue isolation (Fig. 53). Healon®5, Healon® GV, Microvisc® (Plus), Morcher Oil® (Plus), Viscorneal® (Plus) (identical to Allervisc® (Plus) in content), and other viscoelastic substances are considered suitable to counter a flattened anterior chamber, widen a small pupil, simplify a complicated capsulorhexis, resolve synechiae, or counter iridal and vitreous prolapse (Fig. 54). Endothelial dystrophy (Fuchs Dystrophy, advanced cornea guttata), torn posterior capsule or vitreous prolapse are particularly well suited for Viscoat® application (followed by: AMO® Vitrax®, HPMC Ophta® H, Visco Shield™, and other HPMC products). These viscoelastics are preferred substances in case of zonular dialysis with vitreous body prolapse or sinking nucleus (Fig. 55).

The employment of Viscoat® to open fibrotic capsular bags, separate capsule segments and reposition decentralized silicone IOLs with plate haptics, was seen to be of use (Fine & Hoffman, 1997).

Healon5, Microvisc Plus, Healon GV, Visko Plus, Viscorneal (Allervisc) Plus, Microvisc, Dispasan (Ophthalin) Plus, Viscorneal, BioLon Prime, Healon, BioLon, Provisc, Visko, Dispasan, Amvisc, HYA-Ophtal	Viscoat, AMO Vitrax, HPMC Ophta H, Visco Shield, LA GEL, other HPMC products

stabilization/movement   *selective* **isolation/movement**

• shallow anterior chamber • difficult capsulorhexis • small pupil • synechia/adhesion • iris prolapse/vitreous pressure	• compromised corneal endothelium (cendothelial dystrophy, cornea guttata) • hole in the posterior capsule • vitreous prolapse in zonular dialysis • lift nucleus

Fig. 53. Selection of the most suitable viscoelastic substance based on the kind of preoperative situation or intraoperative complication (tissue stabilization versus selective tissue isolation), modified according to Arshinoff 1999, personal communication

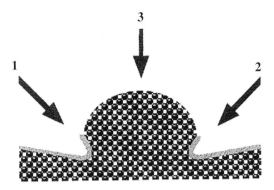

Fig. 54. Selective movement and pushback of the vitreous by injection of a dispersive viscoelastic substance in case of a tear in the posterior capsule with vitreous prolapse and intact vitreous humor membrane (best case scenario):
1. The viscoelastic substance is injected sideways coming from the outside and pointing towards the center of the capsular tear. The edge of the capsular tear is pushed backwards
2. The initial injection around the capsular lesion followed by an injection on the top of the prolapse ensures a backward movement of the vitreous (instead of a possible drift sideways)
3. The vitreous humor is completely repositioned into the vitreous slightly behind the level of the posterior capsule. The use of a viscous viscoelastic substance with longlasting space maintaining capability is recommended to stabilize this situation and to counteract a repeated vitreous prolapse (e.g., during IOL implantation)

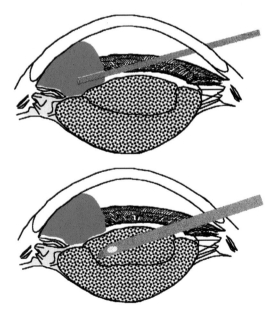

Fig. 55. Selective tissue isolation by the application of a dispersive viscoelastic substance in case of a circumscript zonular dialysis:
1. The viscoelastic is applied at the area of zonular dialysis first. Because of its rheological characteristics the viscoelastic will stay at the application site
2. Phacoemulsification can be continued after injecting a viscous viscoelastic of high and longlasting space maintaining efficiency, thereby minimizing lens movement and tractive forces to the zonular fibers

CHAPTER 6

Complications Through the Use of Viscoelastics

Viscoelastic material retained behind the IOL may cause a capsular bag distension in the early postoperative period. These eyes accumulate a transparent substance in the closed chamber inside the capsular bag from the IOL blocking the capsular opening. The capsular bag distension was first discribed by Davison in 1990. Miyake et al. proposed a new classification of capsular block syndrome and supposed viscoelastic material to cause early-postoperative capsular block syndrome (Miyake et al., 1999). Capsular bag distension after optic capture of a sulcus-fixated IOL was described by Basti et al. (1999).

Complications from the use of viscoelastic substances occur either as a result of improper injection (e.g., overfilling) or incomplete removal.

The principal drawback of viscoelastic use is their propensity to raise intraocular pressure, particularly when residue remains in the eye (Naeser et al., 1986; Olivius & Thornburn, 1985). In the test group where OVD (Viscoat®) was not removed from the anterior chamber following phacoemulsification, more cases of elevated intraocular pressure postoperatively were seen, than were seen in the test group from which OVD was removed (Probst, Hakim & Nichols, 1994). The average increase was seen as higher in the un-aspirated group but without statistical significance (Probst, Hakim & Nichols, 1994). A different study conducted by Stamper, DiLoreto & Schacknow (1990) demonstrated no differences in early postoperative intraocular pressure (with and without aspiration) with use of hyaluronic acid (Amvisc®) in ECCE.

The molecular size of viscoelastics protects from diffusion. Viscoelastics pass out of the eye through the trabecular meshwork as a large, usually unchanged molecule (Berson, Patterson & Epstein, 1983). As contractile elements are present both within the trabecular meshwork and ciliary body, this process is probably dynamic (Balazs, 1983). Several rabbit studies prove that sodium hyaluronate is carried away by both the episcleral veins as well as the mucoscleral pathway, followed by hyaluronidase break down within the tissues (Iwata, Miyauchi & Takehana, 1984; Iwata & Miyauchi, 1985; Miyauchi & Iwata, 1984, 1986).

Numerous factors lead to trabecular obstruction caused by viscoelastics: viscosity, molecular volume, chain length, molecular rigidity and molecular charge (Denlinger, Schubert & Balazs, 1980b; Denlinger & Balazs, 1989; Levy & Boone, 1989). Trabecular pore sizes vary. A variety of prostaglandins, as well as other inflammatory substances, released in response to surgery and trauma (alteration in the blood-aqueous barrier), are also believed to exert an influence over trabecular obstruction. Viscoelastic substances possibly drive fibrin and inflammatory cell-breakdown-products into the chamber angle. In primary open angle glaucoma, a glycosaminoglycan overload of the trabecular meshwork is thought to take place (Tofukuji, 1994). Further overload contributes to the already compromised canals with the occasional development of very high intraocular pressure. Following ECCE, without viscoelastic, postoperative intraocular pressure in eyes suffering from primary open angle glaucoma was seen to be significantly higher than in eyes without other known pathological disturbances (besides cataract) (Barak et al., 1996).

In cadaver eyes, sodium hyaluronate lessened aqueous outflow. Irrigation did not restore outflow facilities. Subsequently injected hyaluronidase was, however, effective in animal and human studies (Barany1956; Calder & Smith, 1986; Lang, Mark & Miller, 1984).

Glasser and co-workers (1986) injected 0.4 ml of different viscoelastic substances into cat eyes through a 3 mm limbal incision and determined intraocular pressure after viscoelastic retention and subsequent removal. All 4 viscoelastic substances presented with the highest intraocular pressure values 2 hours following removal, while 8-24 hours later, pressure was restored close to pre-operative values. Within the aspirated group, significantly lower intraocular pressure values were measured than the non-aspirated group, and the phase of raised intraocular pressure was of shorter duration. These results correspond with a plethora of animal experiments and clinical trials (Fig. 56), which also displayed raised intraocular pressure in the early postoperative phase (Glasser, Matsuda & Edelhauser, 1986; Gross et al., 1988; MacRae et al., 1983; Schubert, Denlinger & Balazs, 1984). These authors all highlight the relevance of 4-8 hour postoperative pressure measurements, particularly in eyes with advanced glaucoma damage,

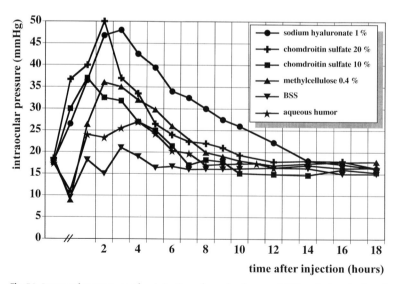

Fig. 56. Intraocular pressure after injection of equal volumes of different viscoelastic substances and control substances into the anterior chamber of rabbits (slightly modified according to Mac Rae et al., 1983)

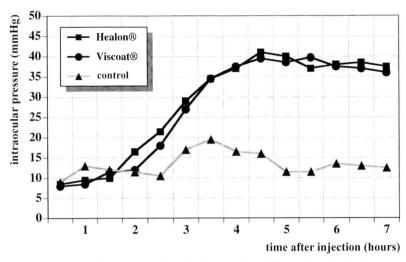

Fig. 57. Intraocular pressure after injection of equal volumes of two different viscoelastic substances into the eyes of monkeys (modified according to Miller, 1989)

likely to worsen if allowed to experience raised postoperative intraocular pressure (Hayreh, 1980; Savage et al., 1985).

Miller (1989) led comparative studies on intraocular pressure after injection and retention of Healon® and Viscoat® into monkey eyes (Fig. 57). Seven monkeys were injected (through a paracentesis) with Healon® into one eye and Viscoat® into the other. Two monkeys served as controls, receiving physiological saline solution. Intraocular pressure was measured pneumatonometrically at 30 minute intervals. Maximal values were noted between 4 and 6 hours later, with intraocular pressure normalizing after 24 hours.

Many other prospective, randomized clinical studies using various hyaluronic acid viscoelastic substances revealed similar postoperative intraocular pressure results, (Anmarkrud, Bergaust & Bulie, 1992, 1995 and 1996; Baron et al., 1985; Colin et al., 1995; Embriano, 1989; Fry, 1989; Gaskell & Haining, 1991; Kohnen, von Ehr & Schütte, 1995; Lehmann et al., 1995; Özmen et al., 1992; Øhrstrøm et al., 1993; Sharpe & Simmons, 1986). Kammann and co-workers (1991) found no statistically significant difference when comparing Healon® and Adatocel® following phacoemulsification.

Early postoperative increases in intraocular pressure were seen to differ, however, between various hyaluronic acid-containing viscoelastic substances in ECCE procedures (Henry & Olander, 1996). In a prospective, blind, randomized study, Fry and Yee (1993) found a significantly raised intraocular pressure 8 hours following ECCE with application of Healon® GV (higher concentration as well as molecular weight) with respect to Healon®. A similar difference was not manifest with phacoemulsification (Kohnen et al., 1996).

Glasser and co-workers regarded the highest possible removal of viscoelastic substance from the eye as a prophylactic measure against raised postoperative intraocular pressure (1986; Fig. 58).

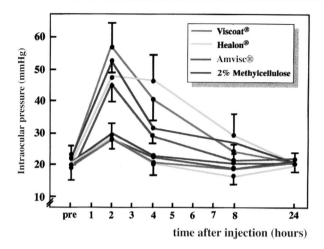

Fig. 58. Intraocular pressure after injection of equal volumes of different viscoelastic substances in eyes of cats. Upper graphs: without the aspiration of the viscoelastic substance; Lower graphs: with the aspiration of the viscoelastic substance (modified according to Glasser et al., 1986)

Therapy for Raised IOP Following Phacoemulsification

Although the mechanism of postoperative pressure increase following viscoelastic application has not yet been elucidated, the hypothesis suggesting an obstruction of the trabecular meshwork caused by the relatively large viscoelastic molecules is largely accepted (Berson et al., 1983; Passo et al., 1985). Attempting to remove the viscoelastic from the anterior chamber as thoroughly as possible diminishes the probability of postoperative intraocular pressure increase. Prophylactic treatment with local and systemic antiglaucomatous medications present a possibility to avoid acutely raised intraocular pressure, in the immediate postoperative phase. Kanellopoulos and coworkers (1997a) compared 60 eyes in a prospective randomized study administering both timolol (gel form; 1 drop Timoptic XE®, protracted effect) and acetazolamide (500 mg Diamox Sequels®) prophylactically, directly following phacoemulsification, and again later the same evening. The average intraocular pressure in eyes pretreated with timolol (15.9 mmHg) was statistically significant lower than the acetazolamide-treated eyes (19.5 mmHg) on the first postoperative day. It was concluded that the prophylactic use of locally applied timolol gel was more effective and showed less side-effects than oral acetazolamide in reducing viscoelastic induced intraocular pressure peaks. Three different surgeons, however, were involved in this trial and operation-time, trauma and the change in the blood-aqueous barrier were not examined. Furthermore, 6 eyes with glaucoma were included in the study, 3 of which demonstrated an intraocular pressure of > 25 mmHg in the acetazolamide group. As all eyes exhibiting intraocular pressure of greater than 25 mmHg resulted in the acetazolamide group, the authors associate this outcome with possible low patient compliance with oral intake.

As treatment for postoperative pressure peaks, acetazolamide (Lewen & Insler, 1985), as well as diverse beta-blockers (Duperre et al., 1994; Fry, 1992; Kanellopoulos et al., 1997a and b; Percival, 1982; Pfeiffer, 1993) and parasypathomimetics (e.g., pilocarpine) have been shown to lower intraocular pressure to varying extents.

Concomitant hyaluronidase administration with OVD lead to improved drainage and protected the eye from rises in pressure (Hein, Keates & Weber, 1986).

CHAPTER 7

Special Uses of Viscoelastics

Viscoelastics have broad clinical applications:
- Cataract surgery
- Corneal surgery
- Glaucoma surgery
- Trauma surgery
- Posterior segment surgery
- Surgery of eye muscles
- Lacrimal surgery[1]
- Lacrimal dysfunction (coating medium)

Cataract, corneal and trauma surgeries particularly necessitate viscoelastic application.

Cataract Surgery

Routine

Viscoelastics are useful for several routine steps involved in cataract surgery:
- Coating the corneal endothelium for protection against lens particles and irrigation fluid
- Pushing back the vitreous and iris-capsule diaphragm to maintain a deep anterior chamber
- Protection against small iris-prolapse and its repositioning
- Dilatation of the pupil (viscomydriasis) as well as its maintenance
- Moving the anterior capsule segment and keeping it from curling up
- Hydraulic loosening of anterior or posterior synechiae
- Hydraulic separation of nucleus and cortex
- Supporting nuclear rotation in capsular bag
- Lens expulsion[2] (i.e., the lens cortex) by injection under the lens capsule[3]

---

[1] Lerner & Boynton, 1985
[2] Stegmann & Miller, 1982
[3] Friedburg, 1994

- Filling up and extending the capsular bag, the ciliary sulcus or the chamber angle for intraocular implantation
- Coating the IOL

The possibilities of viscoelastic use in phacoemulsification will be outlined in the following figures.

Many ophthalmic surgeons apply viscoelastic substances in capsulorhexis to achieve a deep anterior chamber and extend the pupillary space (with a small pupil). Care must be taken during injection so that aqueous is permitted to flow out. When using a paracentesis to inject viscoelastic (Fig. 59), it must be big enough to allow aqueous outflow. For complete aqueous exchange in the anterior chamber, it is advisable to inject the viscoelastic into the opposite chamber angle.

Storage recommendations are to be followed carefully: physicochemical characteristics are preserved through proper storage (hyaluronate must be kept cool! – except for AMO Vitrax® and Rayvisc®). Vials should be kept upright in order to allow air to collect in the injection tip and be removed prior to use. Different preparations demonstrate a substantial amount of air bubbles (Fig. 60), while others do not. Should air bubbles be transmitted with a viscoelastic (Fig. 61), capsulorhexis could be substantially hindered (Fig. 62).

With homogenous filling of the anterior chamber with viscoelastic (Fig. 63), no diffractions, etc., occur. Should the capsulorhexis be performed with a forceps allowing a controlled movement of the capsule in all three dimensions, a larger bulbar opening would be required (Fig. 64) compared to a rhexis performed by a needle. High viscosity at rest (zero shear rate viscosity) hinders the exit of viscoelastic out of the incision site normally associated with the flattening of the anterior chamber. Furthermore, a high viscous viscoelastic maintains chamber depth dependent on the relaxation time.

Low cohesive and good coating viscoelastics (Fig. 65) offer desirable endothelial protection during the actual phacoemulsification procedure (Fig. 66) and from the subsequent irrigation and aspiration maneuver (Fig. 67) without prematurely rinsing out.

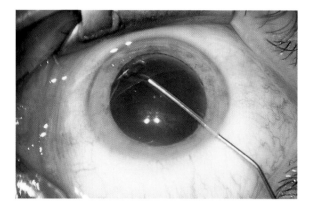

Fig. 59. Injection of a viscoelastic substance via a paracentesis

Fig. 60. New vials with viscoelastic substances: The top
product contains no air bubbles at all. The middle product houses one air bubble,
while the bottom product dis-
plays two air bubbles (at both
ends of the syringe)

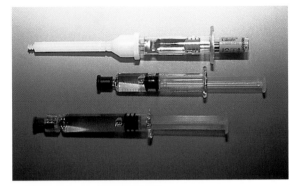

Fig. 61. Viscoelastic substance
in the anterior chamber with
entrapped bubbles of air (see
text)

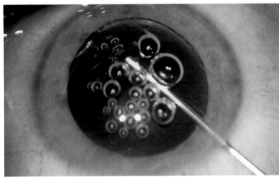

Fig. 62. Air bubbles deriving
from the viscoelastic product
may hinder the view during
capsulorhexis

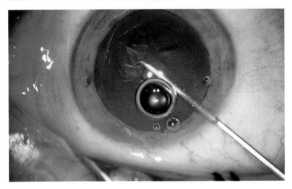

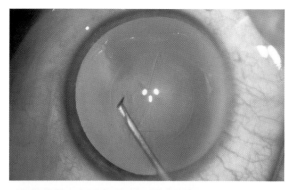

Fig. 63. A homogenous filling of the anterior chamber provides a clear sight during capsulorhexis using a manually bent needle (26-gauge, Sterican, Braun, Melsungen, Germany)

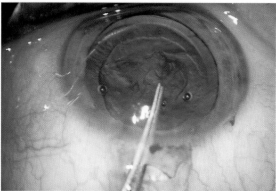

Fig. 64. Capsulorhexis using a superfine capsulorhexis forceps (Geuder, Heidelberg, Germany): a high viscosity at rest prevents an unwanted outflow of the viscoelastic substance

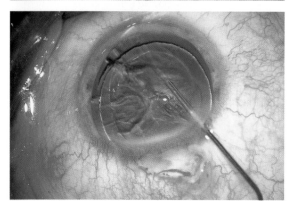

Fig. 65. Injection of a low cohesive well coating viscoelastic substance prior to the phacoemulsification maneuver

Following the polishing of the capsule, viscoelastic is injected to unfold and extend the capsular bag (Fig. 68) thereby occupying space to facilitate intraocular lens implantation.

Following lens implantation, a thorough removal of viscoelastic is advised (Fig. 69, also compare Chapter 8, Aspiration of Viscoelastic).

Fig. 66. Protection of the corneal endothelium by a viscoelastic substance during phacoemulsification

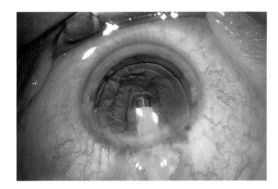

Fig. 67. Bimanual aspiration of cortical remnants using the Schmack I/A device (opening of the irrigation port: 0.5 mm; opening of the aspiration port: 0.3 mm; Geuder, Heidelberg, Germany)

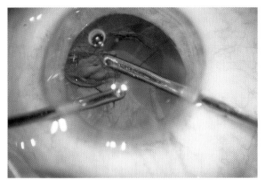

Fig. 68. Injection of a high viscous viscoelastic substance through a small incision to maintain the anterior chamber prior to IOL implantation

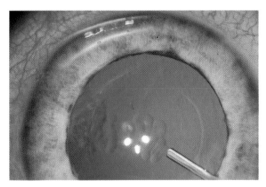

Fig. 69. Bimanual aspiration of the viscoelastiv substance using the Schmack I/A device after IOL implantation

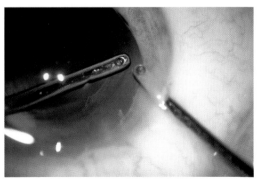

Complications and Difficult Situations

Under complicated conditions viscoelastics particularly facilitate:
- Sealing of bleeding vessels (e.g., iridal or incisional)
- Selective tissue immobilization (e.g., iris; Fig. 70) for specific surgical procedures (e.g., sphincterotomy, iridotomy)[4]
- Tamponading of a port to oppose leakage of air, aqueous or vitreous
- Holding back choroidal bleedings
- Repositioning and treatment of Descemet membrane detachment[5]
- Selective sealing of posterior capsular tears, for a certain duration of time, until completion of nuclear- and cortical- removals
- Tamponading posterior capsule tear for proper positioning of IOL
- Facilitating capsulotomy in mature cataracts with fluid lens material
- Pushing back the vitreous (i.e., anterior vitreous membrane) in primary and secondary IOL implantation, removal or exchange
- Suture placing for IOL fixation
- Anterior chamber maintenance during repositioning of a dislocated IOL
- Capsular bag dissection (e.g., for re-centering IOL)[6]
- As a surgical instrument for anterior chamber-, posterior chamber-, or iris clip-lens removal
- Driving back and protecting the anterior vitreous membrane, in posterior capsulotomy and in secondary cataract dissection[7]
- Cataract extraction in pediatric eyes[8]

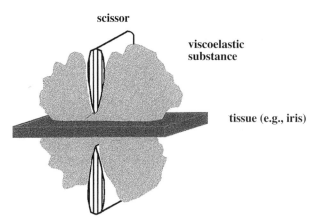

Fig. 70. Tissue mobility (i.e., iris) is reduced by embedding the tissue in viscoelastic substance. This effect is independent on the scissor position. Short microscissor blades can be used, because forward shifting is neutralized

---

[4] Steuhl, Weidle & Rohrbach, 1992
[5] McAuliffe, 1982
[6] Mandelcorn, 1995
[7] Weidle, Lisch & Thiel, 1986
[8] Gimbel et al., 1993; Menezo, Taboada & Ferrer, 1985

Exemplary applications of viscoelastic substances are in cases of mature cataract with liquefied lens cortex (compare Fig. 71). Should the mature lens be intumescent, high viscosity viscoelastic substances in the anterior chamber could supply the counter-pressure necessary to avoid, at least to a certain extent, an uncontrolled tearing of the anterior lens capsule, during capsulotomy (assuming that pressure within the lens capsule is not too high, since no one can possibly perform a capsulorhexis on a blown up, taught balloon). By driving back the milky-white, liquefied lens contents, viscoelastics, by virtue of their transparency, can achieve better optical conditions.

Röver (1995) offers suggestions as to courses of action in dealing with sunken lens nuclei during phacoemulsification; Toczolowski (1987) proposes means of elevating subluxated lenses; and Apple and co-workers (1989) describe IOL exchange with viscoelastic use.

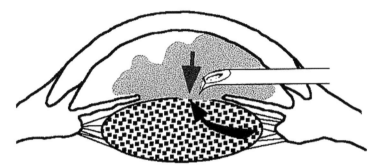

Fig. 71. Viscoblockade may preserve capsular tension and maintain pressure in the capsular bag in case of a mature cataract with liquefied lens: The viscoelastic substance is placed over the capsulorhexis/capsulotomy to keep the liquefied lens contents from escaping. Visualization of the lens capsule is faciliated and bad vision condition which are likely to appear when liquefied lens material mixes up with the aqueous humor is prevented

"Soft -shell" Technique

Steve Arshinoff first introduced the "soft-shell" technique in 1996 (Arshinoff, 1999). This technique was developed with the intention of benefiting both low- and high-viscosity viscoelastic use, as well as minimizing their disadvantages when individually used in phacoemulsification. The first phase of the "soft-shell" technique involves the injection of low viscosity viscoelastic (e.g., Viscoat®) into the pupillary region, forming a small depot-bulge on the lens surface (Fig. 72). The higher viscosity viscoelastic (Provisc®) is then slowly injected into the center of the low viscosity viscoelastic, causing it to spread out and form an even layer, especially under the corneal endothelium (Fig. 73). Under these conditions of fostered anterior chamber stability (impossible to achieve with low viscosity viscoelastic application alone), the capsulorhexis can be performed. The higher viscous viscoelastic leaves the anterior chamber relatively early in the phacoemulsification procedure, while the low viscous viscoelastic remains as a protective, transparent layer (with as few diffraction zones as possible, thereby providing the surgeon with unimpeded visibility) on the corneal endothelium (Fig. 74). The second phase of the "soft-shell" technique involves positioning/extending (Fig.75)

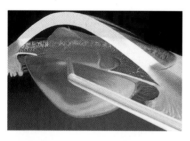

Fig. 72. Injection of the lower-viscosity dispersive viscoelastic agent (violet) into the central region of the pupil to form a mound on the surface of the center of the cataractous lens

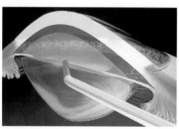

Fig. 73. Injection of the higher-viscosity cohesive agent (green) into the posterior center of the lower-viscosity dispersive viscoelastic agent: continued injection pushes the dispersive agent upward and outward, finally pressurizing it into a smooth protective layer against the corneal endothelium

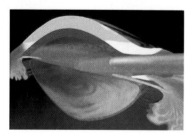

Fig. 74. The higher-viscosity cohesive agent (green) rapidly leaves the eye during phacoemulsification. The smooth layer of the lower-viscosity dispersive agent (violet) will be left to serve as a protection for the corneal endothelial cells

the capsular bag with high viscous viscoelastic (e.g., Provisc®), followed by low viscous viscoelastic injection into the middle of the high viscous viscoelastic (Fig. 76). The low viscous viscoelastic in the anterior chamber facilitates the introduction of instruments and IOL implantation, because of the low resistance of the viscoelastic (Fig. 77). The high cohesive property of the higher viscous viscoelastic, constituting the outside layer, eases the complete removal of viscoelastic at the end of the procedure (Fig. 78). Duo Visc®, a combination of 0.35 ml Viscoat® and 0.4 ml Provisc®, is sold commercially for this particular application.

Criticisms of the "soft-shell" technique include: the relatively large amount of viscoelastic substance used in the first phase, which might possibly account for a shortage later in the course of the operation, and the possibility of low viscous viscoelastic remaining behind the IOL, which would not be easy to aspirate, in the second phase.

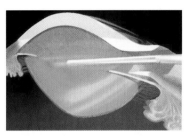

Fig. 75. After removal of the nucleus and cortex the viscoelastic substances are injected in reverse order: the higher-viscosity cohesive agent (green) is injected first. It will occupy the perimeter of the anterior chamber to stabilize the iris, capsule, and anterior chamber depth

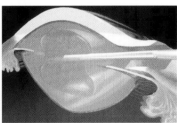

Fig. 76. The lower-viscosity dispersive agent (violet) is then injected into the center of the higher-viscosity cohesive agent by placing the cannula tip approximately in the center of the capsulorhexis

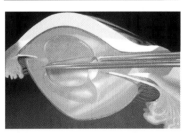

Fig. 77. Presence of the lower-viscosity dispersive agent (violet) in the center of the higher-viscosity cohesive mass (green) allows freer movement of the incoming IOL through the lower-viscosity dispersive agent, with better stabilization of the surrounding iris and capsular bag by the higher-viscosity cohesive agent

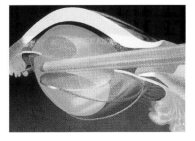

Fig. 78. Both viscoelastic substances are easily aspirated from the eye together at the end of the procedure, because the lower-viscosity dispersive agent (violet) is enveloped within the higher-viscosity cohesive agent (green)

"Best of Both Worlds" Technique

This technique was first described by Thierry Amzallag in an attempt to avoid the above mentioned "soft-shell" technique disadvantages. Here, a low viscous visco-elastic substance (e.g., Viscoat®) is first injected (Fig. 79), followed a by a thin layer of high viscous viscoelastic underneath the low viscous layer, above the lens (Fig. 80). In this way, the capsulorhexis can be performed, covered by high vis-cous viscoelastic, showing high pseudoplasticity (Fig. 81). Although the high vis-cous viscoelastic leaves the anterior chamber during phacoemulsification, the low viscous viscoelastic remains there in a higher proportion (Fig. 82). Before IOL implantation, the higher viscous viscoelastic is injected into the capsular bag (Fig. 83) and then the low viscous viscoelastic is spread thickly on top of it and beneath the corneal endothelium (Fig. 84). This reduces the likelihood that low viscous viscoelastic ends up behind the IOL after implantation (Fig. 85). At the end of the operation, both viscoelastic substances are aspirated; the high viscous viscoelastic from the capsular bag and from above the IOL, and the low viscous viscoelastic from the posterior surface of the cornea (Fig. 86).

The essential differences between this and the "soft-shell" technique are: that each phase consists of two, instead of three viscoelastic layers, that the supposed-ly more effective endothelium-protective low viscous viscoelastic covers the endothelium in each phase; and that IOL implantation subsequently occurs com-pletely within the viscoelastic with higher zero shear rate viscosity and higher pseudoplasticity.

Fig. 79. Injection of the lower-viscosity dispersive viscoelastic agent (violet) into the anterior chamber (like in the dispersive-cohesive viscoelastic soft shell technique)

Fig. 80. Injection of the higher-viscosity cohesive agent (green) on the lens surface and underneath the lower-viscosity dispersive viscoelastic substance

Fig. 81. Capsulorhexis underneath a higher-viscosity cohesive agent (green)

Fig. 82. Phacoemulsification under protection of a lower-viscosity dispersive agent (the higher-viscosity cohesive viscoelastic substance was aspirated at an earlier stage)

Fig. 83. Injection of a higher-viscosity cohesive viscoelastic substance into the capsular bag and partly into the anterior chamber

Fig. 84. Injection of the lower-viscosity dispersive viscoelastic substance (violet) underneath the corneal endothelium above the higher-viscosity cohesive viscoelastic substance (green)

Fig. 85. IOL implantation into the capsular bag

Fig. 86. Aspiration of both viscoelastic substances

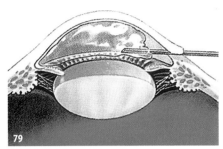

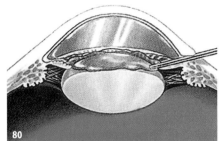

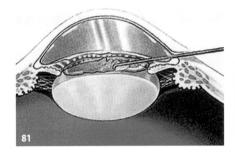

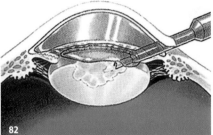

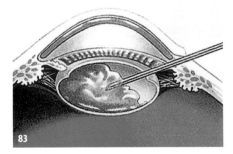

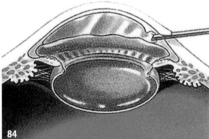

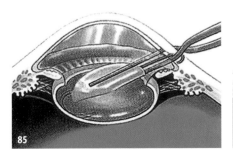

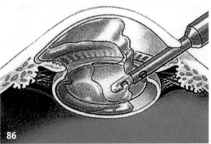

Implantation of Foldable IOLs

The manual implantation of foldable lenses (Fig. 87) is substantially facilitated by and less complicated with a deep, stable anterior chamber and an evenly extended posterior capsule. For introduction of the folded IOL into the capsular bag (Fig. 88), IOL positioning before unfolding (Fig. 89) and the controlled unfolding in the capsular bag, viscoelastic substances of high viscosity and elasticity at low shear rates (e.g., Healon® GV) should be applied. Following implantation, aspiration (Fig. 90) is more easily achieved with cohesive viscoelastic substances than with disperse viscoelastics.

Insertion using an injector (shooters or unfolders) requires a viscoelastic as well, however with other specifications. A small contact angle allows for good coating of the cartridge (Fig. 91) and the foldable IOL (Fig. 92). During injection (Fig. 93), high pseudoplasticity or low viscosity with high shear rates are required

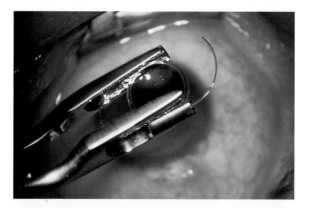

Fig. 87. Foldable multifocal silicone IOL (SA-40N, Allergan, Irvine) in the prefolder (H.-R. Koch universal prefolder forceps, Geuder, Heidelberg, Germany)

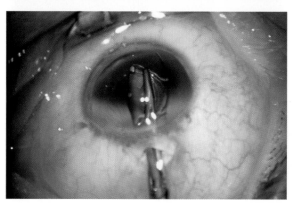

Fig. 88. Implantation of this foldable silicone IOL (before IOL rotation) into the capsular bag using the folding forceps (Geuder, Heidelberg, Germany)

Fig. 89. Implantation of the foldable IOL into the capsular bag (before unfolding starts) using the folding forceps (Geuder, Heidelberg, Germany)

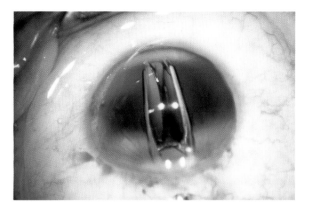

Fig. 90. Aspiration of the viscoelastic substance with an angled I/A tip (Geuder, Heidelberg, Germany) after implantation of a multifocal IOL (SA-40N, Allergan, Irvine, USA)

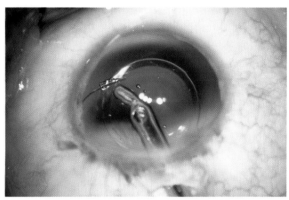

to keep the lens from dragging along the inner surface of the injector. Through folding of the lens within the cartridge (Fig. 94), considerable force builds up because of the high viscosity and shear rates, potentially leading to ripping of the cartridge casing (Fig. 95, 96) or the IOL (Fig. 97). In the meantime, various injector systems are commercially available. The instructions for use given by the manufacturer should be followed, which will reduce the frequency of cartridge crack (Sing et al. 1998; Dick et al. 1999; Olson 1999; Rath et al. 1999).

The unfolding of the IOL in the capsular bag presents the same set of viscoelastic requirements as seen with manual foldable IOL implantation.

A coating OVD with high shear rates permits a more controlled unfolding of the IOL (Fig. 98).

Viscoelastics are employed to coat acrylate lens optics during the folding process (whether to be manually implanted or via injection) to prevent the lens optics from sticking in the folded position.

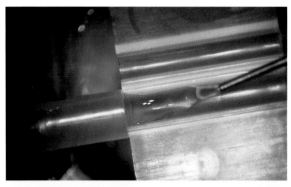

Fig. 91. Preparing the cartridge of the AMO® Phaco-Flex II® implantation system (Unfolder™, Allergan, Irvine, USA): the viscoelastic substance is applied into the tube and in a line along both sides of the through

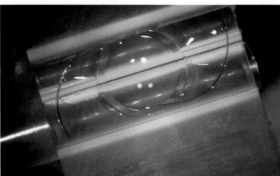

Fig. 92. The IOL is placed into the cartridge, pushed down on the upper and lower edges of the optic to place the optic and loops under the ledges of the cartridge. Then the wings of the cartridge are closed, while the leading loop extends into the cartridge tube

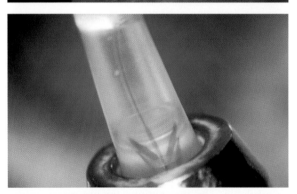

Fig. 93. When the eye is prepared to receive the IOL, the handpiece is gently pushed forward and the leading loop in the cartridge becomes visible. The tube is filled with viscoelastic substance, which can be seen because of a little air bubble on the left side of the leading haptic (detail)

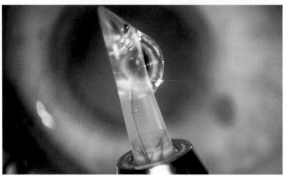

Fig. 94. Overview (see fig. 93)

Fig. 95. Split in the wall of a stretched cartridge tube at the end of the tube after using a low-pseudoplasticity high viscosity viscoelastic substance (light microscopy)

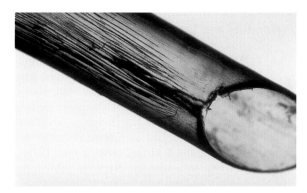

Fig. 96. Longitudinale split in another injector system called Passport (PS-30, Bausch & Lomb, USA) at the opening area with a tangled plate-haptic silicone IOL (Chiroflex C11UB, Bausch & Lomb, USA) also after the correct application of a low-pseudoplasticity high viscosity viscoelastic substance

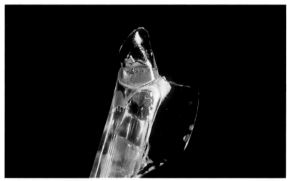

Fig. 97. Tear in the silicone optic (haptic insertion area) after implantation using an implantation system

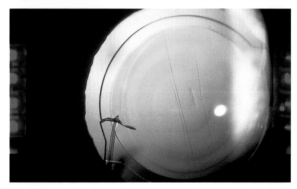

Fig. 98. The IOL is released into the capsular bag under viscoelastic protection

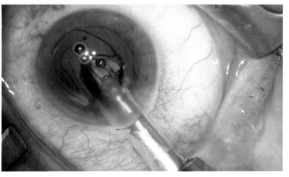

Perforating and Lamellar Keratoplasty

Alpar (1984) observed a reduced endothelial cell loss (10.1%-12.2%) in various penetrating keratoplasty procedures performed with Healon® vs. a 19.4%-20.2% cell loss in the controls. The protective viscoelastic effects on the endothelium and cornea when used in keratoplasty, have been corroborated in a multitude of other studies, as well (Miller & Stegmann, 1981; Polack et al., 1981; Polack, 1982).

Viscoelastics are applied at precise stages of keratoplasty (Severin & Hartmann, 1984; Stegmann & Miller, 1981). Insler (1985) advocates the introduction of viscoelastic (Healon®) into the trephine prior to preparing the donor corneas. Viscoelastic injection into the anterior chamber prior to trephination reduces the risk of damage to underlying tissues and allows the possibility of a regular cut transplant edge (Gruber et al., 1984).

Trephination of an eye with penetrating corneal injury is facilitated by viscoelastic application into the anterior chamber (Maguen et al., 1984). Following removal of the recipient cornea, it is particularly helpful to build up a viscoelastic depot (dome) until a uniform surface is formed. The depot functions as a support (or cushion) upon which the donor corneal endothelium stabilizes and can be adjusted (compare Fig. 99). Positioning of the donor cornea is thus more easily accomplished. The agent also opposes any dislocation of the donor corneal disc into the anterior chamber (Steele, 1983). High viscous hyaluronic acid-containing agents at a higher concentration (Healon® GV) were superior to the low viscous viscoelastic (Healon®) in stabilizing the anterior chamber (Völker-Dieben, Regensburg & Kruit, 1994).

A particular risk involved in perforating keratoplasty is retained viscoelastic in the anterior chamber resulting from the absence of an additional chamber access through which satisfactory aspiration can be performed. A cohesive agent could possibly be rinsed out of the anterior chamber while suture tension is low. Viscoelastic should be bimanually irrigated through 2 separate paracenteses for certainty. A massive rise in IOP may otherwise follow (Schwenn & Pfeiffer, 1997). The formation of "Glaukomflecken" on the anterior capsule can form as a consequence of intraocular pressure decompensation (compare Fig. 100).

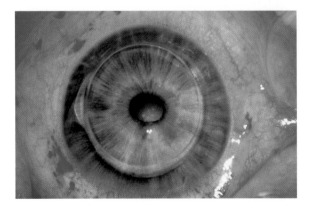

Fig. 99. A viscoelastic pillow in the anterior chamber serves as deposit for the donor cornea in the trepanation opening

Fig. 100. "Glaukomflecken"
at the anterior lens capsule
due to high postoperative
intraocular pressure after
perforating keratoplasty
(1st day postoperatively)

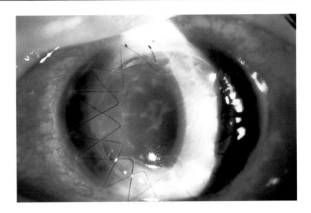

In a randomized study, comparable IOP rises following perforating keratoplasty procedures with OVD retention using Healon® and Viscoat® were noted. Pressure regulation in the Healon® group occurred later (Burke, Sugar & Farber, 1990).

A new surgical technique for deep stromae anterior lamellar keratoplasty was recently described using viscoelastic agents to separate the anterior corneal lamellar (Meller et al., 1999).

Glaucoma Surgery

Since its introduction, trabeculectomy has become the most common fistula-creating procedure in the surgical treatment of glaucoma (Cairns, 1968; Watson, 1970; Watson & Barnett, 1975). One of the advantages of this procedure is its comparatively low incidence of chamber flattening (5–10 %) or collapse (2-4 %), contrasted with for example iridencleisis (24 %) or Scheie-type operations (37 %; Scheie, 1962; D'Ermo, Bonomi & Duro, 1979; Zaidi, 1980). The flattened or collapsed anterior chamber in trabeculectomy plays an important role in the mechanism of cataract formation. 60% of cataracts appearing within the first 6 months following trabeculectomy show a shallow or collapsed anterior chamber (Mills, 1981). The ability of medium viscous hyaluronic acid to occupy the chamber space for a certain duration of time postoperatively and maintain it inspires hope of less postoperative chamber flattening, with the use of this agent in trabeculectomy. Pape and Balazs (1980) examined 15 patients following trabeculectomy using Healon® and concluded that OVD facilitates the procedure, maintaining cameral space in all cases except one. Blondeau (1984) confirmed similar results, suspecting that viscoelastic agents clog the trabecular meshwork allowing aqueous to flow out of the trabeculectomy, keeping it open. Wilson & Lloyd (1986) analyzed the use of Healon® in a large study, including 119 trabeculectomies, without significant differences in postoperative IOP and visual acuity in the Healon® group versus the control group. The rate of postoperative hyphemata in the viscoelastic group was distinctly reduced compared to controls (3 % vs. 20 %). Both Hung (1985) and Raitta and co-workers (1994) established no significant difference in the incidence of postoperative cameral flattening or hypotony between Healon® treated eyes and control groups in a randomized controlled clinical trial of 29 eyes with trabeculectomies. Hung reasoned the absence of the expected viscoelastic effect as possibly due to the thinning and washing out of the OVD by aqueous on the third postoperative day, perhaps through the trabeculectomy fistula. Wand (1988), Charteris & co-workers (1991) and Barak and co-workers (1992) expressed the impression that a sustained deep anterior chamber could be achieved through the intraoperative injection of viscoelastic.

A survey of members of the American Glaucoma Society determined that viscoelastics are used for anterior chamber reformation at the slit-lamp in the postoperative clinical management. Some 47 % used viscoelastic substances in cases of iris-cornea touch, 88% in cases of lens-cornea touch (Salvo et al, 1999).

Charteris and co-workers (1991) observed the formation of thin-walled filtration blebs with more microcysts than in the controls following subconjunctival and subscleral application of 1 % sodium hyaluronate.

Barak and co-workers (1992) pointed out a lower degree of endothelial cell loss after trabeculectomy and an increasing number of postop IOP peaks with sodium hyaluronate use.

In addition to trabeculectomies (Alpar, 1986; Raitta & Setälä, 1986), other surgical glaucoma procedures profited from viscoelastic use, such as goniotomy (especially in congenital glaucoma), cyclodialysis and goniosynechiolysis, due to improved visibility through creation and maintenance of space; e.g., tamponading and spreading of the chamber angle (Wirt, Bill & Draeger, 1992), through separation of tissues (to avoid early adherence of loosened layers) and through hemostatic effect (via tamponade to avoid possible bleeding) (Alpar, 1985; Arnoult et al., 1988; Campbell & Vela, 1984; Draeger et al., 1983; Klemm et al., 1995).

Other surgical techniques endeavor to achieve an adequate pressure sinking effect, either without opening the globe or without creating subconjunctival fistulas. Stegmann propagated viscocanalostomy, which is not an externally fistulating procedure in the true sense of the word (Stegmann et al, 1999). Following the preparation of a sclerocorneal lamella, the roof of the canal of Schlemm is opened and a special cannula is inserted into the canal. Healon® GV is then used for viscodilatation (compare Fig. 101). Viscoelastic injection widens the canal between 30 µm and 150 µm according to Stegmann.

Concomitant preparation of the Descemet's membrane (central to the Schwalbe's line) combined with a deep sclerectomy (actually a deep sclerocornectomy) leads to the formation of a small aqueous pool in the scleral sheath which empties

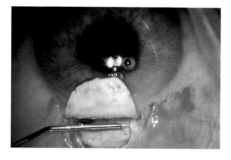

Fig. 101. After dissection of a lamellar sclerocorneal flap and a second flap inside the border of the initial flap (differing in shape) the canal of Schlemm is revealed and un-roofed. A high viscosity viscoelastic substance is then gently injected into the canal. Commonly this procedure will be combined with a deep sclerectomy (the inner scleral flap has already been removed to create an intra-scleral lake)

Fig. 102. In deep sclerectomy a sclerocorneal flap is removed (white area). The deep corneal stroma is removed up to the limbal region creating an intact window in Descemt's membrane. The trabecular meshwork and the canal of Schlemm are un-roofed. The supraciliar space is covered by a very thin scleral layer (light microscopy)

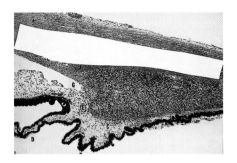

into the dilated canal of Schlemm. The aqueous drainage by-passes the trabecular meshwork, alternatively passing through the water-permeable Descemet membrane directly into the canal of Schlemm. Fig. 102 shows a schematic representation of deep sclerectomy.

In 158 out of 195 eyes (145 patients) with primary chronic open angle glaucoma, intraocular pressure was reduced from a preoperative average of 45 mmHg to a postoperative average of 17 mmHg (after an observation period of 6-45 months), which corresponds to a pressure decrease of 62 % (Stegmann, personal observation, 1998). In 37 eyes, postoperative pressure values could not be reduced to below 23 mmHg. Pressure reductions to values below 23 mmHg were achieved in 82 % of black African patients and in 90% of whites.

The authors wish to add that the combined deep sclerectomy and viscocanalostomy can lower IOP by means of other mechanisms as well. The injection of high viscous viscoelastic into the canal of Schlemm could partially tear the trabecular meshwork thereby reducing drainage resistance, such as seen in trabeculotomy. The application of OVD in the canal and the sclerocorneal space (created as a result of the deep sclerectomy) could hinder hemorrhages into these spaces, thereby contributing to the formation of new postcanalicular trans-scleral drainages, preserving the function of the existent aqueous drainage veins.

Stegmann employs Healon® GV to tamponade the canal of Schlemm and the deep sclerectomy space. Lately, hyaluronic acid implants (SKGEL®35, Corneal, Paris, France) or pork collagen (CGDD 10®, STAAR Surgical, Monrovia, Ca., USA) with longer persistence have been produced.

We described a new dry, cross-linked hyaluronate (Fig. 103a-c) which can be cut exactly to size and replaces the deep scleral flap (Schwenn et al., 1998).

Viscoelastic agents developed from hyaluronic acid are also applied, for instance to keep subconjunctival tissue gaps open in fistula-forming procedures. The rationale behind this measure is to inhibit cell systems. Sodium hyaluronic acid impedes myelo-lymphatic cell membrane movement (Balazs & Darzynkiewisz, 1973), both the direct-chemotactic and random migration of lymphocytes, granulocytes and mononuclear phagocytes (Forrester & Wilkinson, 1981), the phagocytotic activity of macrophages and granulocytes, the transformation and cell division of lymphocytes (Darzynkiewsz & Balazs, 1971), as well as, the in-vitro growth of vascular endothelia as part of the reticuloendothelial system (Raymond & Jacobson, 1982). Growth and cell migration of fibroblasts and epithelial cells are not influenced by the OVD.

In this respect, sodium hyaluronic acid exerts an anti-inflammatory effect which would be likely to slow down or completely arrest the movement and activity of myelo-lymphatic cells from promoting tissue adhesions.

In addition, Balazs (1984) contends that prostaglandin release be held back as well.

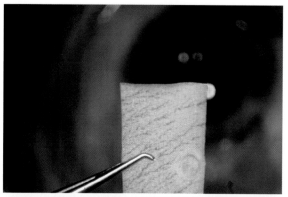

Fig. 103a. Dry crosslinked hyaluronate for deep sclerectomy (Bohus BioTech AB, Strömstad, Sweden)

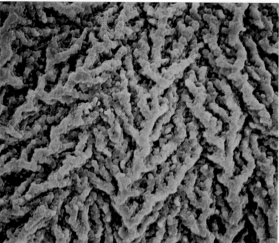

Fig. 103b. Scanning electron microscopy of the hyaluronate implant (magnification × 700)

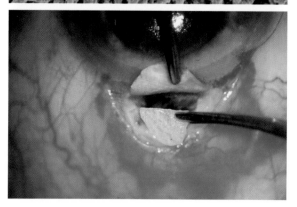

Fig. 103c. The implant is cut to size and replaces the deep scleral flap

Sodium hyaluronate is applied in the treatment of postoperative ocular hypotony in glaucoma surgery. Ocular hypotony caused by overfiltration (Fig. 104) is not only relevant in the development of visual acuity (Schwenn et al., 1996) but also subject to numerous complications. Sodium hyaluronate is particularly well suited for treatment of shallowed anterior chambers (Fig. 105) with threatening lentocorneal contact.

The injection of this agent into a collapsed anterior chamber is a therapeutic possibility (see above; Juzych et al., 1992). Fourman (1990) claims that the above-mentioned OVD application is unsuccessful because of ist short duration of action.

Yet the authors feel the use of high viscous cohesive viscoelastics to be appropriate in inhibiting the threat of corneal injury. Prevention of hypotony and recognition of potential causes (e.g., outward fistula-formation) are of superior significance.

The intravitreal injection of Healon® is also recommended in severe postoperative hypotonia and choroidal hemorrhage (Baldwin et al., 1989; Cadera et al., 1993).

Furthermore, OVD are used topically following 5-fluorouracil application for corneal epithelial care.

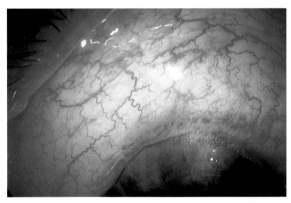

Fig.104. Exuberant bleb formation with excessive outflow after filtering glaucoma surgery

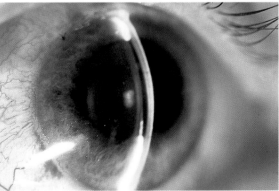

Fig. 105. Flattening of the anterior chamber and threatening lentocorneal contact in case of excessive outflow after filtering glaucoma surgery

Trauma surgery

Viscoelastic agents are highly rated surgical aids for the treatment of perforating bulbar injuries due to their anterior chamber stabilizing and tissue separating properties, decidedly contributing to a better overview at the operation site.

Further references: Bartholomew, 1987; Brown & Benson, 1989; v. Denffer & Fabian, 1984; Drews, 1986; Hirst & DeJuan, 1982; Lemp, 1982; Maguen et al., 1984; Miller & Stegmann, 1982; Rashid & Waring, 1982; Roper-Hall, 1983; Sholiton & Solomon, 1981; Stegmann & Miller, 1986.

Posterior Segment Surgery

The application of viscoelastic substances in posterior segment surgery has largely been relegated to a part of their history. Their usability has faded in the face of new endo-tamponading agents (e.g., gases, perflorcarbons, silicone oils).

Further references: Balazs, 1960; Balazs et al., 1972; Balazs & Hutsch, 1976; Brown & Benson, 1989; Crafoord &Stenkula, 1993; Denlinger & Balazs, 1980; Dunn et al., 1969; Folk et al., 1986; Gerke et al., 1984; Kirkby & Gregor, 1987; Kishimoto et al., 1964; Koster & Stilma, 1986 a and b; Landers, 1982; Lewis et al., 1996; McLeod & James, 1988; Mori, 1967; Müller-Jensen, 1974; Oosterhuis et al., 1966; Poole & Sudarsky, 1986; Pruett et al., 1972; Scott, 1983; Scuderi, 1954; Stenkula et al., 1981; Stenkula, 1989; Stenzel et al., 1969; Swartz & Anderson, 1984; Vatne & Syrdalen, 1986; Verstraeten et al., 1990; Winter, 1987.

Surgery of Eye Muscles

Viscoelastics have also found application in the surgery of the outer eye muscles.

Further references: Clorfeine & Parker, 1987; Ferreira et al., 1995; and Searl et al., 1987.

Lacrimal Dysfunction (Coating medium)

Due to their long transit time on the corneal surface, dispersive HPMC products with a small contact angle are particularly useful intraoperatively for epithelial coating. Intraoperative implementation of hyaluronic acid-containing agents was described for coating use as contact gel, especially for operations with long durations (Federman, Decker & Grabowski, 1983; Norn, 1981). In an examination of epithelial toxicity brought about by OVD use, HPMC-containing products were best tolerated (Linquist & Edenfield, 1994). Furthermore, there are several hyaluronate mixtures which can be used in tear dysfunctions.

Our own mixture is:

sodium hyaluronate eye drops 0.1%	
sodium hyaluronic acid (Serva 25125)	0.01 g
Liquifilm® eye drops for dry eye syndrome	ad 10 ml
sodium hyaluronate ointment 0.2%	
sodium hyaluronic acid (Serva 25125)	0.01 g
phosphate buffer solution	1.5 g
Adeps lanae anhydr.	0.1 g
Ungt. ophthalm. simpl.	
DAC 1986	ad 5.0 g

Mixtures of several different sodium hyaluronate concentrations are commercially available (Vislube®/Vismed®: 0.18%; Laservis®: 0.25%; Hylo-COMOD®: 0.1% Chemedica, München, Germany; Ursapharm, Saarbrücken, Germany).

Chemical burn therapy also makes use of viscoelastics. In the treatment of bacterial corneal ulcers hyaluronic acid has been sucessfully employed as well (Gandolfi, Massari & Orsoni, 1992).

Further literature: Algawi et al., 1995; Chung et al., 1996; DeLuise & Peterson, 1984; Hamano et al., 1996; Imkamp et al., 1988; Limberg et al., 1987; Mengher et al., 1986; Nelson & Farris, 1988; Polack & McNiece, 1982; Reed et al., 1987; Reim & Saric, 1989; Sand et al., 1989.

CHAPTER 8

Removal of Viscoelastic Substances

All viscoelastics should be completely removed from the eye to reduce the likelihood of increased intraocular pressure. Should OVD retention behind the IOL occur, an unstable refraction could result. Residual high molecular viscous substance is transported away through the trabecular meshwork, with delay, possibly resulting in a protracted postoperative IOP increase. To aspirate viscoelastics various techniques as well as instruments with different aspiration/irrigation adjustments have been proposed, a few of which will be described here. Viscoelastic removal involving the simultaneous irrigation and aspiration through a single cannula (Nevyas, 1987) or two separate cannulas (Brauweiler, 1996) is considered to be less traumatic for the corneal endothelium due to the reduced possibility of cameral collapse than earlier methods (involving initial aspiration of the anterior chamber with subsequent chamber reshaping).

Highly viscous agents are removed with more difficulty and were associated with increased early-postoperative intraocular pressure in some studies (Laurell & Philipson, 1995). A high aspiration setting is advised when aspirating high viscous viscoelastics. Aside from positioning the aspiration/irrigation handle in the middle of the anterior chamber above the center of the lens optic, there are essentially 2 other technique options (Auffarth et al., 1994):

1. The tip of the irrigation/aspiration handpiece is led along the edge of the capsulorhexis/pupil in a circular motion through the 4 quadrants or pushed forward below the lens optic. Viscoelastic is first removed out of one half of the capsular bag and the anterior chamber, then the handle is turned 180° and begins aspiration of the other half (Fig. 106).

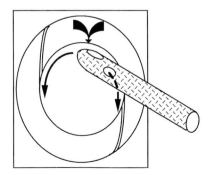

Fig. 106. Aspiration technique: With circling movements the I/A handpiece is gently conducted along the edge of the capsulorhexis or the pupil crossing the four quadrants in the anterior chamber

2. The irrigation/aspiration handle is led beginning from the middle of the IOL radially towards the periphery and turned along the tip axis to release irrigation fluid into the capsular bag (Arshinoff).

Both of these aspiration techniques were shown (in experimental studies on human cadaver eyes) to be especially effective in the almost complete removal of highly viscous agents, compared to the first technique (Auffarth et al., 1994; Wesendahl et al., 1994). After an average of 17 seconds, Healon® and Healon® GV were nearly completely aspirated by a circular motion along the capsulorhexis, while OVD remained in the anterior segment even after 1 minute with the first technique. The shortest removal times were reached (in a closed system) at a high vacuum setting (250 mmHg), with minimal time differences seen between the aspiration of Healon® and Healon® GV (Wesendahl et al., 1994). In an experimental study led by Assia and co-workers (1992) on human post-mortem eyes, distinct differences were seen between complete viscoelastic removal times. While Healon® and Healon® GV were completely removed within 20 and 25 seconds with an automated irrigation/aspiration system, both HPMC preparations and Viscoat® were mostly removed in 1 minute, although completely in about 3 minutes. The type of OVD obviously influences (along with aspiration type and technique) the extent of removal. Hütz and co-workers (1996) stated: "while Healon® was most easily removed from the eye, followed by Healon® GV, the removal of the HPMC product Methocel® (particularly from the chamber angle and behind the IOL) and Viscoat® (particularly from the endothelium and the IOL) was more difficult."

Poyer and co-workers described aspiration kinetics in animal models. Each viscoelastic was aspirated for 2 seconds with increasing vacuum power and then quantified (Fig. 107). It is noteworthy to point out in Figure 107 and Table 14 that different aspiration adjustments were needed to remove different substances.

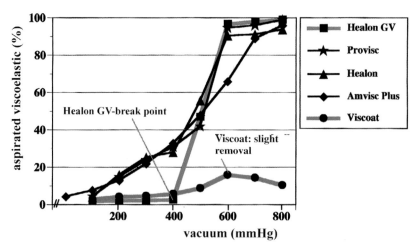

Fig. 107. Aspiration kinetics of different viscoelastics dependent on the vacuum (mmHg); (modified according to Poyer et al., 1998)

Table 14. Break points of various viscoelastic agents (Poyer, Chan, Arshinoff, 1998)

viscoelastic substance	break point* (mmHg)
Healon® GV	381
Provisc®	381
Healon®	381
Amvisc® Plus	254
Viscoat®	no

* The break point (vacuum level at which bolus removal of the agent begins) of a viscoelastic agent is
defined as having more than 25 % of the sample removed by a single vacuum level

Aspiration of Healon® GV was accomplished with higher vacuum than the low
viscous Provisc®, Healon® or Amvisc®. For Viscoat®, no start aspiration value was
given.

The aspiration behavior of HPMC solutions differs from that of hyaluronic
acid solutions and is particularly dependent on molecular weight (Silver et al.,
1993). Low molecular weight HPMC solutions are easier to aspirate than higher
molecular weight solutions (90 000 D) which need a high vacuum adjustment
(Fig. 108). A hyaluronic acid solution with a molecular weight of about 1 Million D
was almost entirely aspirated at certain high-set vacuum gage positions. 90 000 D
HPMC was increasingly better aspirated at higher gage settings. Using HPMC will
probably give postop intraocular pressure rises, as will Healon® and other hyaluronic acids (Liesegang, Bourne & Ilstrup, 1986; Thomsen, Simonsen & Andreassen, 1987).

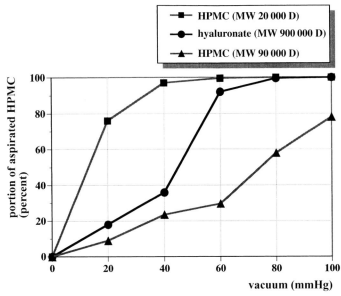

Fig. 108. Aspiration curves of HPMC with different molecular weights and hyaluronate under increasing vacuum conditions ranging from 0 to 100 mmHg (modified according to Silver et al., 1994)

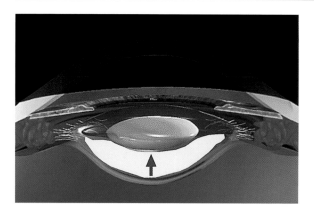

Fig. 109. Remained viscoelastic substance behind the IOL after incomplete removal of the viscoelastic may cause an increase in intraocular pressure postoperatively, a deviation from the target refraction or even a change in refraction

Using fluorescent colors to reveal Healon®, Smith & Burt (1992) observed quicker substance removal and lower incidence of pressure peaks, than without. Blue colored Healon® proved to have an edge in a study designed by Drews (1989).

In a trial performed by Wedrich & Menapace (1992), the removal of viscoelastic from behind the IOL lowered the incidence of early postop intraocular pressure peaks (Fig. 109). To mobilize OVD from behind the IOL, the irrigation/aspiration handle is generally lightly pressed onto the IOL optic. Moving the handle behind the IOL directly should be avoided so as not to aspirate the posterior capsule which would increase the danger of capsular damage (Wesendahl et al., 1994).

Comparison between postoperative intraocular pressures following use of Healon® and Healon® GV was seen in a prospective, randomized study with phacoemulsification and the standard aspiration technique (compare 1) but with 2 different aspiration times (20 vs. 40 seconds), yielding no statistically significant differences (Kohnen et al., 1996). It is much more important, however, to concentrate on the complete and careful removal of viscoelastic agents (especially when aspirating high viscous substances) than on time intervals. In an in-vitro study by Auffarth and co-workers (1994), up to 40 seconds were necessary for the complete removal of, for example, Healon® GV. It therefore seems impractical to recommend any amount of time for the removal of viscoelastics, more so in eyes with glaucomatous damage which are more prone to optic injury resulting from transient IOP peaks.

When removing high viscous agents, cohesion of a large substance mass can give rise to an abrupt motion, which, to be avoided (and to avoid e.g. iridal pigment layer detachment) necessitates an irrigation/aspiration relationship check as well as aspiration power (Hütz et al., 1996).

If the anterior lens capsule edge covers the implant entirely, the possibility of OVD winding up behind the IOL (between it and capsule) is great. The implant can function like a valve, allowing the aqueous to flow behind the IOL, however not allowing the simultaneous exit of OVD. This may cause the implant to press forward. Neuhann suggested the puncturing of the anterior capsule peripherally and next to the optic edge, to allow viscoelastic to escape. If the pupil does not dilate enough, a posterior capsular puncture can be performed to allow viscoelastic to escape into the vitreous. Neuhann stressed, however, that a peripheral puncture may be easier since the central posterior capsule might possibly be displaced far back (Neuhann, 1995).

The "Rock and Roll" Technique

This technique was developed for the specific removal of high viscous viscoelastic, with comparable time and work investment as other methods (Arshinoff). A high irrigation/aspiration phase and flow rate should be set on the phacoemulsification machine. The IOL is pushed slightly downward with the handle, which is briefly left there (Fig. 110). The handle is next rolled to the left to aspirate on one side (Fig. 111) and then rolled to the right to aspirate on the other (Fig. 112). These 2 steps are repeated, slanting the optic from side to side (rock) and circulating the irrigation fluid beneath the IOL optic, for complete removal. Next the irrigation/ aspiration handle is led to make circular movements into the anterior chamber, aspirating from all 4 quadrants (Fig. 113).

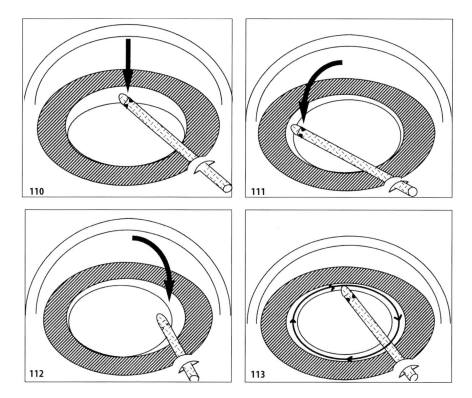

Fig. 110. "Rock and Roll" technique: for viscoelastic removal the IOL is gently pushed down using the I/A tip

Fig. 111. The I/A tip is twisted to the left for aspiration (roll)

Fig. 112. After twisting the I/A tip to the opposite side the aspiration procedure is continued

Fig. 113. Finally, a circling movement is performed with the I/A tip in the anterior chamber. This movement should include all 4 quadrants during the aspiration process

Retention of the Viscoelastic Substance

Factors influencing viscoelastic retention are:
– Dispersive nature (the lower the CDI, Cohesion dispersion index, the higher the retention)
– Negative molecular charge
– Hyaluronic acid receptor sites

Poyer and co-workers (1998) developed a new biological in-vitro model for the indirect, quantitative recording of surface retention on cultivated corneal rabbit endothelial cells vs. retention on a hydrophobic polypropylene surface, following irrigation/ aspiration. The single-cell layer endothelium is dyed. The application of 5 different OVD onto both the polypropylene surface and the cell layer is followed by a 3-minute irrigation/aspiration procedure using 120 ml BSS (with various additives). The fluid turbulence observed is similar to that caused by phacoemulsification. After the use of alcohol to wash the dye out of the cells, which no longer were coated with viscoelastic, the quantity of dye was determined spectrophotometrically. The degree of retention of polypropylene, following the same irrigation/aspiration procedure, was measured with a sensitive scale for weight changes. Retention onto corneal endothelial cells was greater than on polypropylene (Fig.114), which must indicate that factors other than cohesion, such as charge or hyaluronic acid binding-sites, play a role in surface interactions between viscoelastics and endothelial cells. The retention of Healon® and Provisc® on the artificial surface was very low, which suggests that these relatively neutral hyaluronic acid products are more likely to be retained on cell surfaces due to the presence of binding-sites.

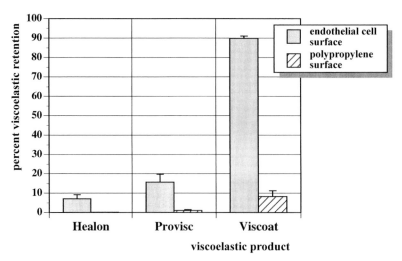

Fig. 114. Percentage of the viscoelastic retention on endothelial cells of the rabbit and on a polypropylene surface after irrigation and aspiration (n=6 up to n=9); (modified according to Poyer et al., 1998)

CHAPTER 9

Healon®5: A New Viscoadaptive Formulation

To relate the practical relevance of our study results, specific requirement profiles for individual procedures have been correlated to the desired physicochemical characteristics. Healon®5 demonstrated the statistically significant highest zero shear viscosity of all OVD and a long relaxation time (Dick et al., 2000). It therefore most effectively creates and maintains a deep anterior chamber in order to facilitate safe surgical maneuvers (e.g., in case of vitreous pressure). Additionally, the high viscosity of Healon®5 exhibits a dynamic frequency dependence, which has not been observed in any pure hyaluronic acid formulation before. Healon®5´s properties change in response to surgical maneuvers. This rheological behaviour possibly reflects the facilitated removal of Healon®5. By means of introducing turbulences and phaco power (continuous high shear rates) creating a high flow situation, Healon®5 becomes less viscous over time by fragmentation. During surgery with high flow situations, it forms a cavity with an outer retentive shell. Healon®5 obtains both, dispersive as well as cohesive characteristics (Fig. 115). In cataract surgery, we recommend the creation of

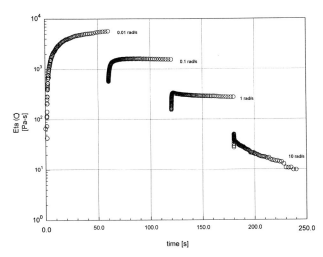

Fig. 115. Dynamic behaviour of the viscosity: At lower shear rates Healon®5 slowly builds up a very high viscosity, whereas at higher shear rates it becomes less viscous. Viscosity further decreases with constant exposure of a certain shear rate = viscoadaptive characteristic

space within the Healon®5 in front of the capsulorhexis before initiating the phacoemulsification to avoid potential complications (e.g., corneal wound burns) due to the innate properties of Healon®5.

The removal of Healon®5 depends on fracturing the molecular mass into smaller pieces, which are free to be aspirated. Therefore, removal is then facilitated especially with the "rock-n-roll" technique first introduced by S. Arshinoff, because the rotation of the irrigation and aspiration tip (anterior chamber turbulence with increased fluid flow rate) shoots fluid waves through the viscoelastic to fracture it. This can be accomplished with standard I/A tip, 0.3 mm, with high settings; flow rate should be 25-30 ml/min, and vacuum 350-500 mmHg, depending on the type of pump. If a peristaltic pump is used the vacuum should be set towards the higher limit. If a venturi pump is used the vacuum should be set towards the lower limit. Bottle hight should be 60-70 cm above eye level. An alternative technique (two compartments technique) has been developed by M. Tetz allowing the use of less turbulance using the same settings mentioned above (Tetz & Holzer, 2000). The removal is started by directly going behind the IOL optic without engaging the flow of the I/A tip and then starting flow, while the anterior chamber is still filled with Healon®5. The tip is then removed from behind the IOL optic while maintaining continuous flow and placed on top of the optic.

In two recent studies, Healon®5 caused statistically significant lower intraocular pressure (IOP) increase and significantly fewer IOP spikes than Viscoat in the early period after small incision cataract surgery (Schwenn et al., 2000). Nevertheless, removal of Healon®5 from the anterior chamber as well as from behind the IOL is necessary at the end of surgery with great care. The removal of the highly viscous Healon®5 took 15 to 60 seconds. Precautions to prevent IOP increase are necessary especially in eyes with an already damaged optic nerve or impairment of the ocular drainage system.

When performing phacoemulsification with topical anesthesia, the outer eye muscles retain their tonus, explaining the absence of a "soft" eye and possibly raised vitreous pressure. Raised vitreous pressure may encumber capsulorhexis or IOL implantation because of a shallowed anterior chamber. Besides high viscosity at zero shear rate, constant space-occupying effectiveness is indispensable in such cases. Some OVDs alter their molecular configuration when experiencing external pressure, even without application of shear force, and thereby also change their viscosity at rest.

The super-viscous cohesive agents facilitated surgical maneuvers and endothelial protection more than viscous cohesive agents. By combination of different properties, Healon®5 combines advantages of cohesive and dispersive properties. From the rheological standpoint it is the most ideal product for each step of the phacoemulsification procedure compared to Healon® and Healon® GV.

CHAPTER 10

Aseptic Production vs. Terminal Sterilization

The safety of substance use in intraocular surgery ideally requires the absence of all biologically-active components capable of causing an inflammatory reaction. Substance purity is achieved with isolation and cleansing methods (e.g., of the polysaccharide), which remove any biological component with infective potential. The methods of production for polysaccharide isolation should remove biological agents, regardless of its origin. Hyaluronic acid is isolated either from rooster combs or biological fermentation. Use of this substance showed the development of postoperative intraocular inflammatory reactions resulting from contaminations from both sources. OVD should have low endotoxin values. Although many manufacturers claim their products to be pyrogen-free, this is hardly ever attained in practice. The lowest acceptable endotoxin concentration of a substance used intraocularly has not yet been established. For some manufacturers, a concentration of up to 3 EU/ml is acceptable. It is in fact not yet clear at which concentration exactly inflammatory reactions occur in mammals. It seems justified to require < 0.5 EU/ml, as is standard for other medicinal products intended for injection into the human body. As increasingly confusing terminologies have been noted up lately, certain terms should be elucidated (Sharp, 1995). The term sterility is defined as the complete absence of living organisms (so-called "Orange Guide", 1983). Sterility is an absolute state; i.e., there is no gradual grading of sterility. Sterile is defined as that which is in the state of sterility (Sharp, 1995). An OVD batch can be sterilized by different methods, however, the probability of a non-sterile particle in the batch is dependent on the method employed. This probability is described as SAL (sterility assurance level) and represents the highest probability of non-sterility of a unit, after the sterilization process.

Terminal sterilization is sterilization through heat or radiation of the product in its final storage form (Fig. 116). For terminally sterilized products, the SAL is 1:1 000 000, or, 1 out of a million units is not sterile, in the best case. Of the examined viscoelastics, only the following are terminally sterilized: Healon®, Healon® GV, Healon®5 (all three: Pharmacia & Upjohn; Sweden), Viscorneal®, Viscorneal® Plus (both: Corneal, Pringy, France), Allervisc®, and Allervisc® Plus (both: Allergan; Ettlingen, Germany).

Another sterilization method is aseptic production, in which the separately sterilized product components are combined under aseptic conditions. According to pharmacopoeia of the USA "the overall efficiency of an aseptic operation and ... the microbial survivor probability of aseptically processed articles" is 1:1000,

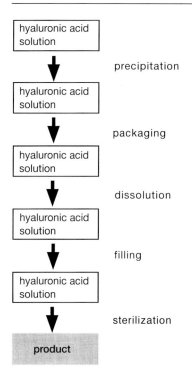

Fig. 116. Production process with terminal sterilization

i.e., maximally 1 non-sterile unit results in 1000. In this context, it is noteworthy to point out that various aseptic production methods are used for viscoelastic products. Some are produced through sterile ultrafiltration in the final production step (the filling step) which is also the only aseptic step in production. Other substances are sterilely ultrafiltrated during different steps: precipitation, drying, dissolving and filling (Fig. 117). It follows that the probability of non-sterile particles varies with production methods as well as the supervision of surroundings: personnel, machines, containers, among other things. Both terminal sterilization and aseptic production are authorized by the responsible administration. In case product integrity is compromised (loss of stability, chemical alteration etc.) by terminal sterilization, it can be aseptically manufactured.

The extent of rheologic weakening through terminal sterilization is largely dependent on a substance's molecular weight. Following terminal sterilization a certain number of glycoside bonds are broken within the polysaccharide resulting in reduced molecular weight and consequently also viscosity. This viscosity reduction could be compensated for by raising the concentration. Hyaluronic acid with a high molecular weight could conceivably be reduced up to 30%, with zero shear viscosity reduction of up to 80%. This reduction could be balanced by a 30% concentration increase. The extent of medium molecular weight hyaluronic acid degradation through terminal sterilization is as high as with a molecule of 10 000 000 D since the number of broken glycoside bonds are

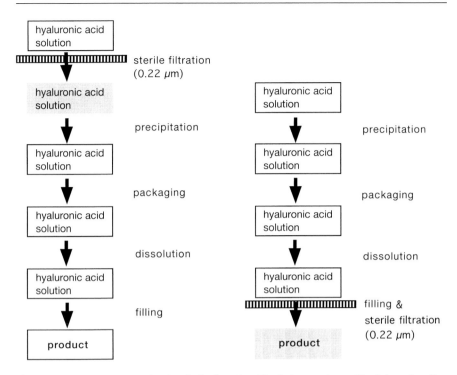

Fig. 117. During its aseptic production the hyaluronic acid solution can be sterilised through a filter (0.22 μm) before the first step of the production process or at the last step (filling). In terminal sterilisation the already filled product is sterilised (e.g., autoclavation)

equal in both. Yet this effect is seen less commonly with hyaluronic acid of medium molecular weight. The lower viscosity (at lower molecular weights) through terminal sterilization is rare, however, and can be ignored for practical purposes.

CHAPTER 11

Viscoelastics: Medical Device or Drug

In § 2 of the German Drug Laws (AMG, Arzneimittelgesetz), it is determined that such materials that fall under the heading of medicinal products (MPG, Medizinproduktegesetz, 1994) are not drugs in the AMG sense of the word. MPG medicinal products, as defined in §3 are those substances whose main effect is neither pharmacological, immunological, nor metabolic.

If one alleges that the main function of viscoelastics is to protect the endothelium, this would only then describe the above stated definition if the effect were achieved through metabolism. This is not the case even when considering endothelial protection through viscoelastics from the aspect of electrolyte-metabolism, if one considers electrolyte metabolism of endothelial cells to be included in the broader sense of metabolism.

The literal interpretation of MPG § 3 supports this view, since regulations require that the effect be reached via metabolism. OVD do not achieve their effects via the metabolism, but merely protect it and contribute to its maintenance at times. The bare maintenance of the metabolism (so-called expanded metabolism notion) does not lead, if taken literally, to substance classification as a drug. This result is supported by the historical interpretation; i.e., the interpretation of the norm according to the will of the legislators. The European legislators must redress guideline 93/42 as it is merely converted from the MPG. In which way the European legislators mean "effect achieved through metabolism" is the reference point of the Borderline-Paper from July, 1995, its continuation from February, 1998, and 2 opinions from Garth Thompson, who worked on guideline 93/42 from 5/10/96 and 2/13/98.

The Borderline-Paper from July, 1995, defines metabolism in this way, that normal chemical processes become altered. The working paper from February, 1998, makes clear that the term alteration include the termination, beginning and change of the speed of normal chemical processes. According to this elucidation, the sole maintenance of metabolism through OVD does not include it as a medicinal product. Both papers from the EU-Working Commission verify a narrow definition of metabolism. The systematic interpretation of § 3 speaks against a material being a drug, or any combination of materials being a drug, if it merely maintains natural metabolism; because the effect achieved via metabolism is equivalent to a pharmacological or immunological effect. According to these definitions, stated by these 2 documents, these modes of action also effect a change in the natural body functions. Even BSS solution, which most closely resembles aqueous fluid and assumes its function, does not alter natural body functions, was categorized as a medicinal product and not a drug, by the courts of Frankfurt in 1998.

CHAPTER 12

Summary

OVD are irreplaceable parts of ophthalmic surgery and are used routinely worldwide in cataract surgery and other surgical anterior segment procedures. Especially in complicated cases, the protective effect, for example, on the corneal endothelium, is unchallengeable. At the moment, the number of commercially available viscoelastic preparations is increasing. They are essentially composed of 3 different basic elements: sodium hyaluronic acid, a mixture out of sodium hyaluronic acid with chondroitin sulfate, and HPMC. HPMC has the advantage of being inexpensive. The multiple sources of HPMC and the many combinations of it give rise to impurities, therefore, one should use reservedly. Some commercial preparations have undergone improvement due to a manufacturing procedure including a complicated filtration process, which made a far-reaching purification of the product possible. Human enzymes cannot completely metabolize HPMC and the fate of HPMC residual break-down products in the human body is not completely clear. So far, there are no indications of side-effects from the amounts used. HPMC was not shown to have any toxic effects on the endothelium in animal studies.

The choice of OVD depends on the intended surgical procedure. To maintain the anterior chamber and for tissue manipulation, sodium hyaluronate offers advantages. These result mainly from the high molecular weight, high viscosity at low shear rates, high elasticity and pseudoplasticity. A mixture out of sodium hyaluronate and chondroitin sulfate offers similar properties, although removal from the eye requires increased attention due to adherence of the mixture. It coats tissues and instruments and possibly conducts less drag forces onto the corneal endothelium due to its lower viscosity.

Coatability of the endothelium is only an advantage as long as the OVD has no toxic effects or produces no drag force injuries during aspiration to the endothelium.

When asked about the preferred OVD indication profile, almost 70 % of all US colleagues chose to have a viscoelastic substance for all cases (Leaming, 1998).

Unfortunately, no OVD can fulfill all desired properties at once. The choice of substance should fulfill the operation profile requirement, with less emphasis on the price, and take into account known complications with consideration to the desired physicochemical properties. Arshinoff's grouping of viscoelastics into 2 categories based on company information was modified according to the study results at hand and the wide spectrum of viscoelastic characteristics.

Uniform specifications with regard to chemical, toxic, rheologic and clinical properties by the manufacturers and distributors would be desirable.

Better knowledge of viscoelastics facilitate differentiated selection depending on the preoperative clinical situation and the occurring surgical difficulties.

The authors have no financial or commercial interest in any product or object mentioned in this book.

Appendix

Product Overview

The following information was taken from brochures provided by the individual companies and was confirmed by them in almost all cases. In the case of vacant positions in the tables the companies were either unable or refused to give the proper information.

Table 15. Hyaluronic acid products

Product	AMO Vitrax®	Amvisc®	Allervisc®	Allervisc® Plus	BioLon®	Dispasan®	Dispasan® Plus
Manufacturer	Allergan, West-port, Ireland	Bausch & Lomb, USA	Corneal, France	Corneal, France	Bio Technology General, Rehorot Israel	Ciba Vision Ophthalmics, Germany	Ciba Vision Ophthalmics, Germany
Provider in Germany	Pharm-Allergan, Ettlingen	Bausch & Lomb, Dornach	Pharm-Allergan, Ettlingen	Pharm-Allergan, Ettlingen	Pharma Stulln, Nabburg	Europe: Ciba Vision; Ophthalin	Europe: Ciba Vision; Ophthalin
Substance/ingredients per ml	30 mg sodium hyaluronate 3.20 mg sodium chloride, 0.75 mg potassium chloride, 0.48 mg calcium chloride, 0.3 mg magnesium chloride, 3.9 mg sodium acetate, 1.7 mg sodium citrate	16 mg sodium hyaluronate 9 mg sodium chloride	10 mg sodium hyaluronte 8.5 mg sodium chloride, 0.563 mg disodium hydrogenphosphate, 0.045 mg sodium dihydrogenphosphate, aqua ad injectibila	14 mg sodium hyaluronate 8.5 mg sodium chloride, 0.563 mg disodium hydrogenphosphate, 0.045 mg sodium dihydrogenphosphate, aqua ad injectibila	10 mg sodium hyaluronate sodium chloride	10 mg sodium hyaluronate sodium chloride	15 mg sodium hyaluronte sodium chloride
Concentration (%)	3	1.6	1	1.4	1	1	1.5
Production	rooster combs	bacterial fermentation	rooster combs	rooster combs	bacterial fermentation	bacterial fermentation	bacterial fermentation
Molecular Weight (Dalton)	500 000	1.5 Mio.	5 Mio.	5 Mio.	~3 Mio.	2 Mio.	>3 Mio.
Osmolarity (mosmol/l)	310	331±43	320	320	-	290-350	300-350
Osmolality (mosmol/kgH$_2$O)	-	340	270-390	270-390	258-381	-	-
pH-value	7.3	6.9±0.7	7.0	7.5	6.5-7.5	7.2-7.8	7.2-7.8
Elasticity	-	-	-	-	-	4.49 Pa at 0.01 Hz	-

Table 15 continued

Product	AMO Vitrax®	Amvisc®	Allervisc®	Allervisc® Plus	BioLon®	Dispasan®	Dispasan® Plus
Viscosity (mPa·s)	40 000	60 000±4000	200 000	500 000	–	35 000 (25° C, shear rate 2 sec^{-1})	2 500 000
storage: Δ = avoid exposure to light and freezing	at room temperature 15°–30° C, Δ	2°–8° C, avoid exposure to freezing	2°–8° C, Δ	2°–8° C, Δ	4 weeks at 25° C, 2°–8° C, Δ	2°–8° C, Δ	2°–8° C, Δ
Pack size (ml)	0.65	0.5 and 0.85	0.55 and 0.85	0.55 and 0.85	0.5 and 1.0	0.5 and 1.0	0.5

Table 16. Hyaluronic acid products

Product	Healon®	Healon® GV	Healon®5	Microvisc®	Microvisc® Plus	Morcher Oil®	Morcher Oil® Plus
Manufacturer	Pharmacia & Upjohn, Uppsala, Sweden	Pharmacia & Upjohn, Uppsala, Sweden	Pharmacia & Upjohn, Uppsala, Sweden	Bohus Bio Tech, Strömstad, Sweden	Bohus Bio Tech, Sweden	Bohus Bio Tech, Sweden	Bohus Bio Tech, Sweden
Provider in Germany	Pharmacia & Upjohn, Erlangen	Pharmacia & Upjohn, Erlangen	Pharmacia & Upjohn, Erlangen	Schwagerl, Hanau	Schwagerl, Hanau	Morcher, Stuttgart	Morcher, Stuttgart
Substance/ ingredients per ml	10 mg sodium hyaluronate sodium salt 5000, 8.5 mg sodium chloride, 0.28 mg sodium dihydrogenphosphate, 0.04 mg sodium monohydrogenphosphate, aqua ad injectibila	14 mg sodium hyaluronate sodium salt 7000, 8.5 mg sodium chloride, 0.28 mg sodium dihydrogenphosphate, 0.04 mg sodium monohydrogenphosphate, aqua ad injectibila	23 mg sodium hyaluronate sodium salt 7000, 8.5 mg sodium chloride, 0.28 mg sodium dihydrogenphosphate, 0.04 mg sodium monohydrogenphosphate, aqua ad injectibila	10 mg sodium hyaluronate 1.4 mg disodium-dihydrogenphosphate, 8.3 mg sodium chloride, 0.26 mg potassium dihydrogenphosphate, aqua ad injectibila	14 mg sodium hyaluronate 1.4 mg disodium-dihydrogenphosphate, 8.3 mg sodium chloride, 0.26 mg potassium dihydrogenphosphate, aqua ad injectibila	10 mg sodium hyaluronate 1.4 mg disodium-phosphate-dihydrate, 8.3 mg sodium chloride, 0.26 mg potassium dihydrogenphosphate	14 mg sodium hyaluronte, 1.4 mg disodium-phosphate-dihydrate 8.3 mg sodium chloride, 0.26 mg potassium dihydrogenphosphate
Concentration (%)	1	1.4	2.3	1	1.4	1	1.4
Production	rooster combs	rooster combs	rooster combs	rooster combs	rooster combs	rooster combs	rooster combs
Molecular weight (Dalton)	4 Mio.	5 Mio.	4 Mio.	5 Mio.	7.9 Mio.	6.1 Mio.	7.9 Mio
Osmolarity (mosmol/l)	304	304	304	-	-	-	-
Osmolality (mosmol/kgH$_2$O)	309	302	309	312–370	322–338	312–370	322–338
pH-value	7.0–7.5	7.0–7.5	7.0–7.5	7.0–7.5	7.0–7.5	7.0	7.5
Elasticity	26 Pa at 0.1 Hz	110 Pa at 0.1 Hz	-	-	-	-	-

Table 16 continued

Product	Healon®	Healon® GV	Healon®5	Microvisc®	Micrivisc® Plus	Morcher Oil®	Morcher Oil® Plus
Viscosity (mPa·s)	200 000 (25° C, shear rate 0 sec⁻¹)	2 000 000 (25° C, shear rate 0 sec⁻¹)	7 000 000 (25° C, shear rate 0 sec⁻¹)	-	-	1 000 000	1 000 000
storage: Δ = avoid exposure to light and freezing	2°–8° C, Δ	2°–8° C, Δ	2°–8° C, Δ	2°–8° C, Δ	2°–8° C, Δ	2°–8° C, Δ	2°–8° C, Δ
Pack size (ml)	0.4, 0.55 and 0.85	0.55	0.6	0.55 and 0.85	0.55 and 0.85	0.55	0.55

Table 17. Hyaluronic acid products

Product	Provisc®	Rayvisc®	Viscoat®	Viscorneal®	Viscorneal® Plus	Visko®	Visko Plus®
Manufacturer	Alcon, Fort Worth, USA	Rayner Hove, England	Alcon, Fort Worth, USA	Corneal, Pringy, France	Corneal, Pringy, France	–	–
Provider in Germany	Alcon Pharma, Freiburg	Rayner, Deutschland	Alcon Pharma, Freiburg	Corneal, Mainz	Corneal, Mainz	Domilens, Hamburg	Domilens, Hamburg
Substance/ ingredients per ml	10 mg sodium acid, 0.56 mg sodium monohy-drogenphosphate, 0.04 mg sodium-dihydrogenphos-phate, 8.4 mg sodium chloride hypochloric acid and/or sodium hydroxide, aqua ad injectibila	30 mg sodium hyaluronate, 0.5 mg sodium chloride, 0.056 mg potassium chloride, 0.036 mg calcium-chloride, 0.022 mg magnesium chloride, 0.042 mg disodium hydro-genphosphate, 0.006 mg sodium dihydrogenphos-phate, aqua ad injectibila	A) 40 mg chon-droitin sulfate, sodium salt, B) 30 mg hyalu-ronic acid, sodium chloride, 0.45 mg sodium dihydrogenphos-phate, 2.0 mg sodium monohydrogen-phosphate, 4.3 mg sodium chloride, aqua ad injectibila	10 mg sodium hyaluronate, 8.5 mg sodium chloride, 0.563 mg disodium hydro-genphosphate, 0.045 mg sodium dihydrogenphos-phate, aqua ad injectibila	14 mg sodium hyaluronate 8.5 mg sodium chloride, 0.563 mg disodium hydrogenphos-phate, 0.045 mg sodium dihydro-genphosphate, aqua ad injectibila	10 mg hyaluronic acid, 0.563 mg disodium hydrogenphos-phate, 0.045 mg sodium dihydro-genphosphate, 8.5 mg sodium chloride, aqua ad injectibila	14 mg hyaluronic acid, 0.563 mg disodium monohy-drogenphosphate, 0.045 mg sodium dihydrogenphos-phate, 8.5 mg sodium chloride, aqua ad injectibila
Concentration (%)	1	3	4.3	1	1.4	1	1.4
Production	bacterial fermentation	bacterial fermentation	A) shark fin cartilage B) bacterial fermentation	rooster combs	rooster combs	rooster combs	rooster combs
Molecular weight (Dalton)	>1.1 Mio.	550000–800000	A) 22 500 B) >500 000	5 Mio.	5 Mio.	2 Mio.	3 Mio.
Osmolarity (mosmol/l)	–	–	–	320	320	–	–

Table 17 continued

Product	Provisc®	Rayvisc®	Viscoat®	Viscorneal®	Viscorneal® Plus	Visko®	Visko Plus®
Osmolality (mosmol/kgH$_2$O)	310	320	330	270-390	270-390		
pH-value	7.25±0.25	6.8-7.5	7.25±0.25	7.0	7.5	7-7.5	7-7.5
Elasticity	-	-	-	-	-	-	-
Viscosity (mPa·s)	50000±20000 (shear rate 1 sec^{-1})	50000	30-50 (shear rate 1 sec^{-1})	200000	500000	300000	500000
storage: Δ = avoid exposure to light and freezing	2°-8° C, Δ	2°-30° C, Δ	2°-8° C, Δ	2°-8° C, Δ	2°-8° C, Δ	2°-8° C, Δ	2°-8° C, Δ
Pack size (ml)	0.55 and 0.85	0.85	0.5	0.55 and 0.85	0.55 and 0.85	0.55 and 0.85	0.55 and 0.85

Table 18. HPMC-products

Product	Acri® Visc	Adatocel®	Coatel®	HPMC-Ophtal® L	HPMC-Ophtal® H	LA GEL®
Manufacturer	Acrimed, Glienicke, Germany	Bausch & Lomb, Germany	Chauvin OPSIA, Labége Cedex France	LCA SA, Paris, France	LCA SA, Paris France	LA LABS, USA
Provider in Germany	s. manufacturer	s. manufacturer	Chauvin, Nuremberg	Dr. Winzer Pharma, Olching	Dr. Winzer Pharma, Olching	Domilens, Hamburg
Substance/ingredients per ml	20 mg methyl-cellulosepropyl-glycerolether, sodium chloride, potassium chloride, calcium chloride-2 H_2O, lactic acid, hydrochloric acid, sodium hydroxide	methylhydroxy-propylcellulose 18.0 to 22.0 mg, sodium chloride, potassium chloride, calcium chloride × H_2O, lactic acid, hydrochloric acid, sodium hydroxide, water for injection	20 mg methyl-hydroxypropyl-cellulose, 4.9 mg sodium chloride, 0.75 mg potassium chloride, 0.48 mg calciumchloride, 0.3 mg magnesium chloride, 3.9 mg sodium acetate, 1.7 mg sodium citrate, HCl/sodium hydroxid buffer solvent	20 mg methyl-hydroxypropyl-cellulose, 9 mg sodium chloride, 2.7 mg boric acid, 0.2 mg sodium, aqua ad injectibila	20 mg methyl-hydroxypropyl-cellulose, 9 mg sodium chloride, 2.7 mg boric acid, 0.2 mg sodium, aqua ad injectibila	18 mg hydroxy-propylmethylcellulose, 5.9 mg sodium chloride, 0.75 mg potassium chloride, 0.48 mg calcium chloride, 0.3 mg magnesium chloride, 3.9 mg sodium acetat, 1.7 mg sodium citrate
Concentration (%)	2	ca. 2	2	2	2	1.8
Production	-	synthetic	-	synthetic	synthetic	-
Molecular weight (Dalton)	~86 000	~86 000	>8 500	80 000	250 000	1.3 Mio
Osmolarity (mosmol/l)	283±17	283±17	-	330	330	-
Osmolality (mosmol/kgH$_2$O)	-	-	275-325	-	-	-

Table 18 continued

Product	Acri® Visc	Adatocel®	Coatel®	HPMC-Ophtal® L (low)	HPMC-Ophtal® H (high)	LA GEL®
pH-value	6.2±0.3 (20° C)	6.2±0.3	7.2	7.2±0.2	7.2±0.2	7.2±0.4
Elasticity	–	–	40% between 0.1 and 10 Hz	–	–	–
Viscosity (mPa•s)	4500±400	4500±400	5000±1500	4800 (25° C and shear rate 0.5 sec⁻¹)	55000 (25° C and shear rate 0.5 sec⁻¹)	40000
storage: Δ = avoid exposure to light and freezing	at room temperature	below 25° C	at room temperature	at room temperature	at room temperature	at room temperature
Pack size (ml)	1.5	2.25	1.0 and 2.0	1.5	1.0	1

Table 19. HPMC-products

Product	Ocucoat®	PeHa-Visco®	Visco Shield™
Manufacturer	Storz Ophthalmics, Clearwater, USA	PeHa-Intraokular-linsen, Germany	Storz Ophthalmics, Clearwater, USA
Provider in Germany	Bausch & Lomb, Heidelberg	Halfwassen, Unna	Domilens, Hamburg
Substance/ ingredients per ml	20 mg methyl-hydroxypropyl-cellulose, 0.49% sodium chloride, 0.075% potassium chloride, 0.048% calcium chloride, 0.03% magnesium chloride 0.39%, sodium acetate, 0.17% sodium citrate, aqua ad injectibila	20 mg hydroxy-propylmethyl-cellulose, 6.4 mg sodium chloride, 0.75 mg potassium chloride, 0.48 mg calcium chloride, 0.3 mg magnesium chloride, 3.9 mg sodium acetate, 1,7 mg sodium citrate	20 mg methylhy-droxypropylcellulose, 0.49% sodium chloride, 0.075% potassium chloride, 0.048% calcium chloride, 0.03% magnesium chloride, 0.39%, sodium acetate, 0.17% sodium citrate, aqua ad injectibila
Concentration (%)	2	2	2
Production	derived from natural substances	-	-
Molecular weight (Dalton)	>80 000	-	800 000
Osmolarity (mosmol/l)	285±32	-	275-325
Osmolality (mosmol/kgH$_2$O)	-	313±3	-
pH-value	7.2±0.4	6.97	6.8-7.6
Elasticity			
Viscosity (mPa·s)	4000±1500	2585	40 000
storage: Δ = avoid exposure to light and freezing	at room temperature avoid exposure to light	at room temperature avoid exposure to light	at room temperature avoid exposure to light
Pack size(ml)	1.0	2.0	1.0 and 2.0

Measured Values for Certain Products Gained by Individual Investigations

Individual rheological properties of the investigated viscoelastic products in alphabetical order and subdivided by classes of substances (for specific information about the viscoelastic products see text and tables). The graphs below show the viscosity (Pa sec), the elasticity modulus G' (Pa), as well as the viscosity modul G" (Pa) in dependency of the shear rate.

Viscoelastics Containing Hyaluronic Acid

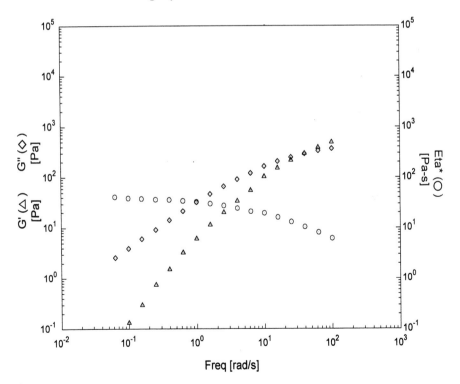

Fig. 118. AMO Vitrax®

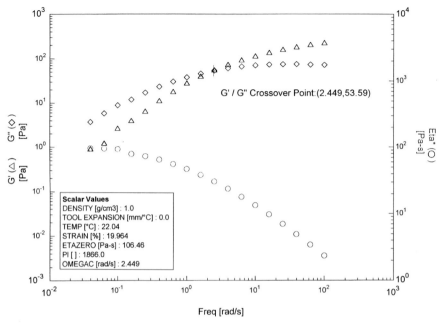

Fig. 119. Amvisc®

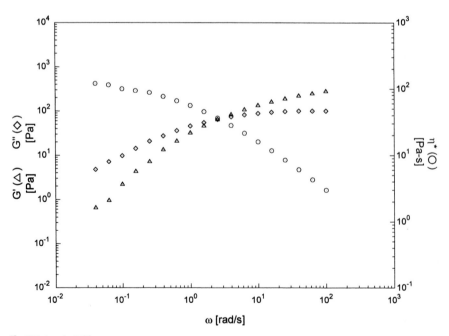

Fig. 120. Amvisc® Plus

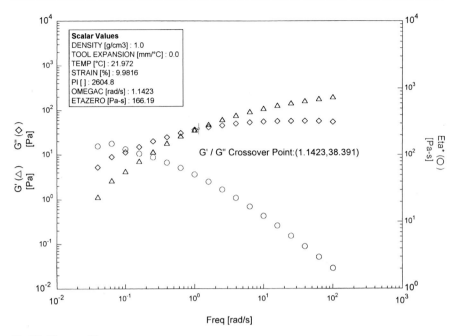

Fig. 121. Biocorneal®

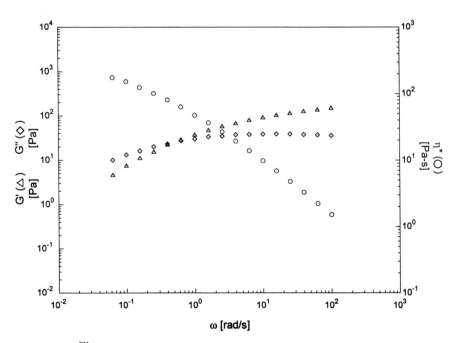

Fig. 122. BioLon™

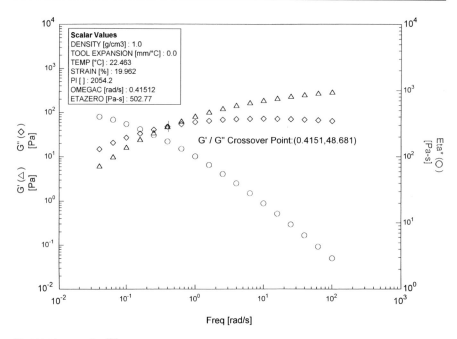

Fig. 123. BioLon Prime™

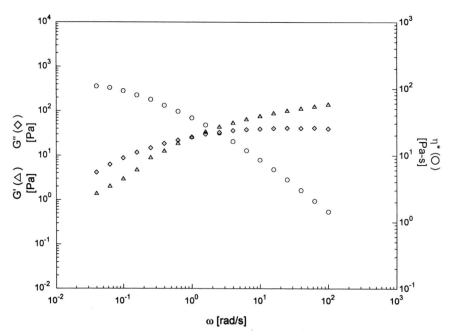

Fig. 124. Dispasan® (Ophthalin®)

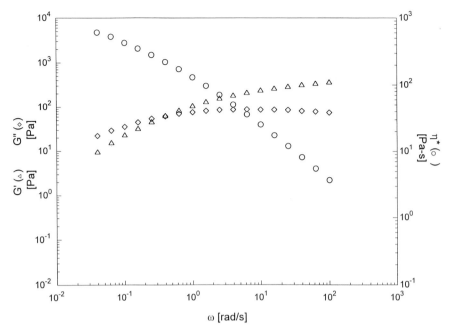

Fig. 125. Dispasan® (Ophthalin® Plus)

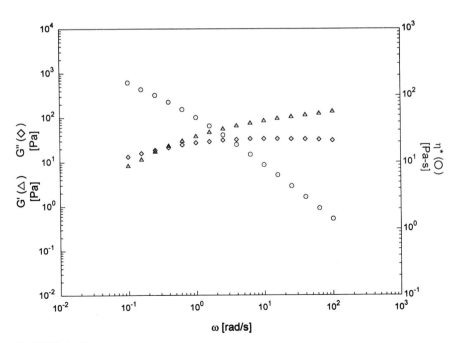

Fig. 126. Healon®

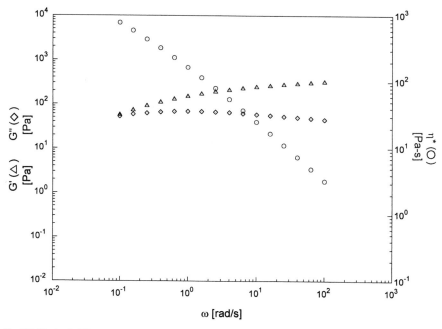

Fig. 127. Healon® GV

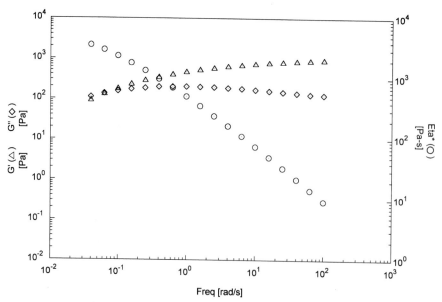

Fig. 128. Healon®5

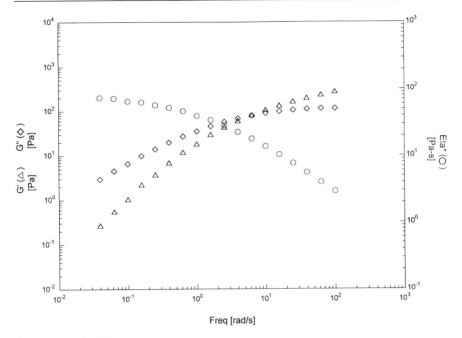

Fig. 129. HYA Ophtal®

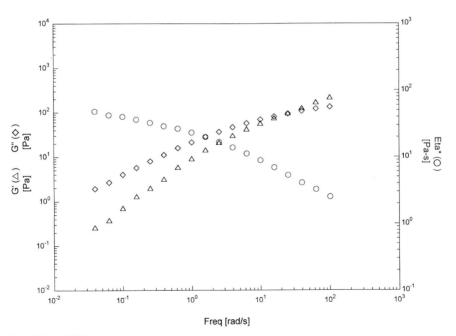

Fig. 130. LA GEL®

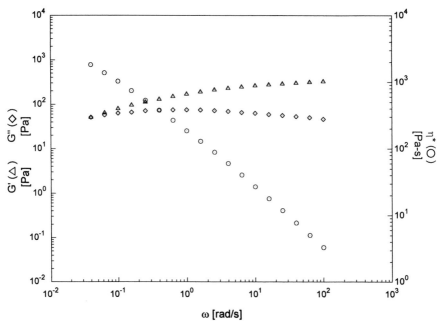

Fig. 131. Microvisc® (Morcher Oil®, HSO®)

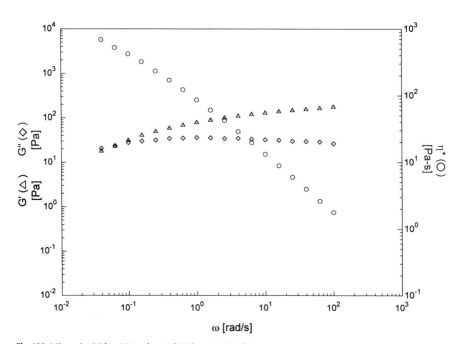

Fig. 132. Microvisc® Plus (Morcher Oil® Plus, HSO® Plus)

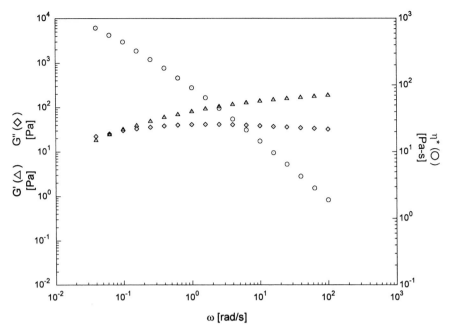

Fig. 133. Morcher Oil® Plus

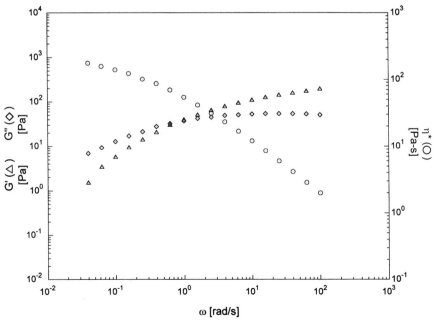

Fig. 134. Provisc®

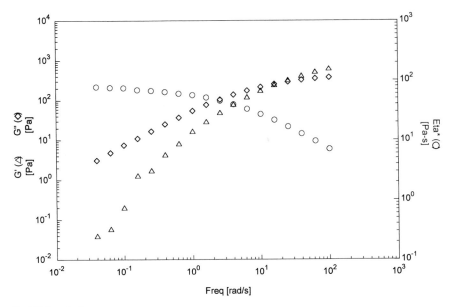

Fig. 135. Rayvisc®

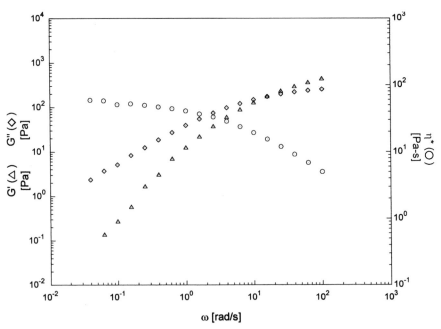

Fig. 136. Viscoat®

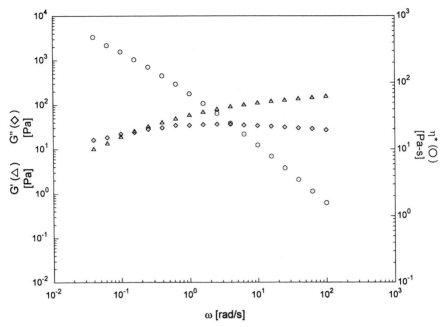

Fig. 137. Viscorneal® (Allervisc®)

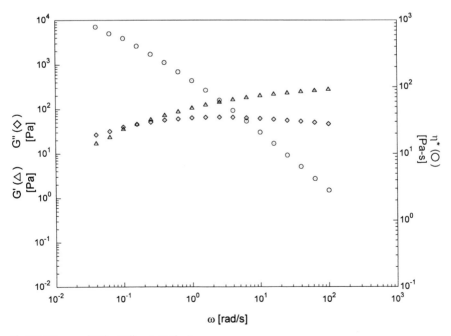

Fig. 138. Viscorneal® Plus (Allervisc® Plus)

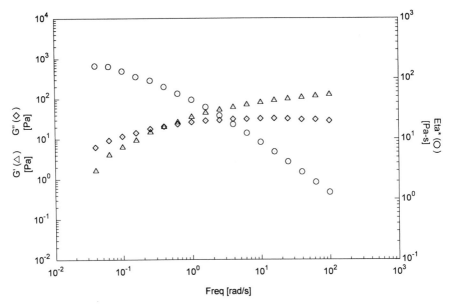

Fig. 139. Visko®

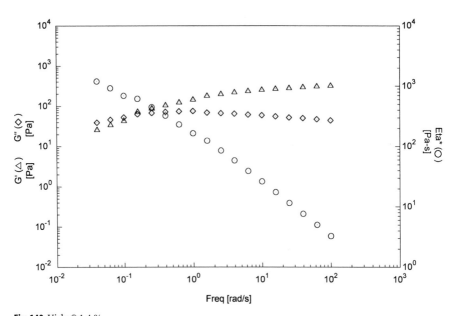

Fig. 140. Visko® 1.4 %

Viscoelastics from Hydroxypropylmethylcellulose

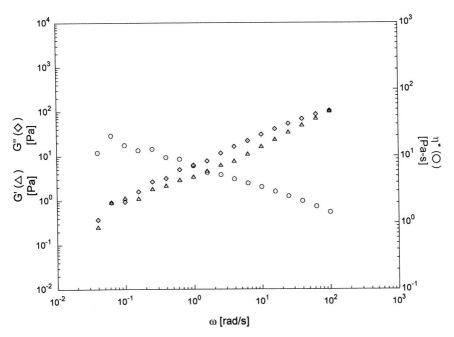

Fig. 141. Acrivisc®

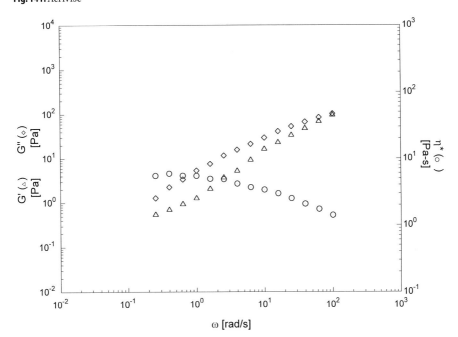

Fig. 142. Coatel®

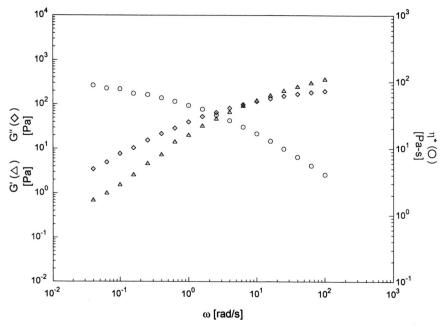

Fig. 143. HPMC Ophtal H®

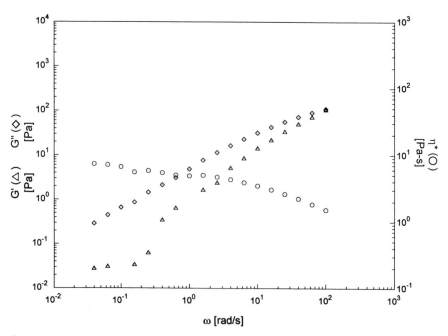

Fig. 144. HPMC Ophtal L®

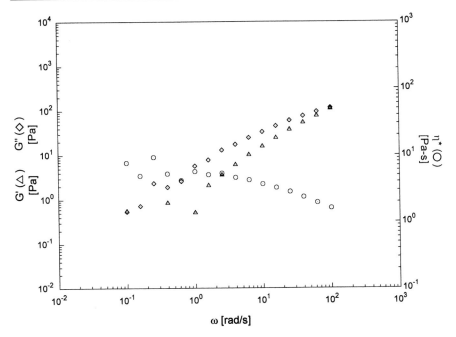

Fig. 145. Ocucoat®

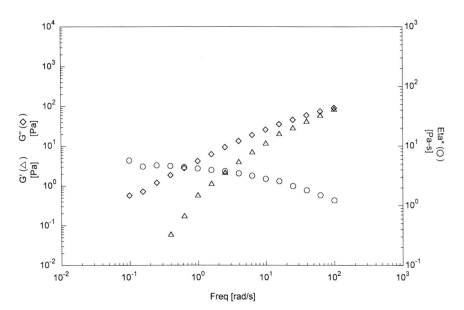

Fig. 146. PeHa-Visco®

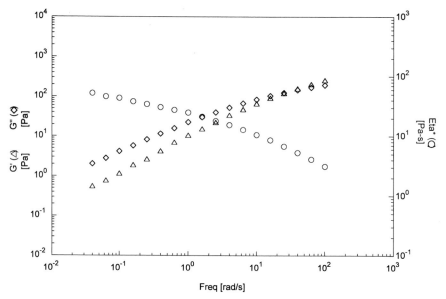

Fig. 147. Visco Shield™

References

Reviews

Alpar JJ. Viscosurgery: a review of materials, indications, techniques and precautions. Eisner G (ed): Ophthalmic Viscosurgery: A Review of Standards, Techniques and Applications. Bern, Switzerland, Medicopea International, 1986, S. 39–53

Buratto L, Giardini P, Belluci R. Viscoelastics in ophthalmic surgery. Thorofare, SLACK Incorporated, 2000

Larson RSL, Lindstrom RL, Skelnik DL. Viscoelastic agents. CLAO J 1989; 15:151–161

Liesegang TJ. Viscoelastic substances in ophthalmology. Surv Ophthalmol 1990; 34:268–293

Meyer-Schwickerath G (Hrsg). Viskochirurgie des Auges. Stuttgart, Enke, 1984

Miller D, Stegmann R. Healon (Sodium Hyaluronate): A Guide to Its Use in Ophthalmic Surgery. New York, John Wiley 35:410–416

References

Algawi K, Agrell B, Goggin M, O'Keefe M. Randomized clinical trial of topical sodium hyaluronate after excimer laser photorefractive keratectomy. J Refractive Surg 1995; 11:42–44

Alpar JJ. The use of Healon in corneal transplant surgery with and without intraocular lenses. Ophthalmic Surg 1984; 15:757–760

Alpar JJ. Comparison of Healon and Amivsc. Ann Ophthalmol 1985; 17:647–651

Alpar JJ. Sodium hyaluronate (Healon®) in cyclodialysis. CLAO J 1985; 11:201–204

Alpar JJ. Sodium hyaluronate (Healon®) in glaucoma filtering procedures. Ophthalmic Surg 1986; 17:724–730

Alpar JJ, Alpar AJ, Baca J, Chapman D. Comparison of Healon® and Viscoat® in cataract extraction and intraocular lens implantation. Ophthalmic Surg 1988; 19:636–642

Anmarkrud N, Bergaust B, Bulie T. The effect of Healon and timolol on early postoperative intraocular pressure after extracapsular cataract extraction with implantation of a posterior chamber lens. Acta Ophthalmol (Copenh) 1992; 70:96–100

Anmarkrud N, Bergaust B, Bulie T. The quantitative effect of Healon on early postoperative intraocular pressure after extracapsular cataract extraction with implantation of a posterior chamber lens. Acta Ophthalmol (Copenh) 1995; 73:537–540

Anmarkrud N, Bergaust B, Bulie T. A comparison of Healon and Amvisc on the early postoperative pressure after extracapsular cataract extraction with implantation of a posterior chamber lens. Acta Ophthalmol (Copenh) 1996; 74:626–628

Apple DL, Tetz MR, Hansen SO, Solomon K. Use of viscoelastics in intraocular lens removal. Rosen ES (ed): Viscoelastic Materials: Basic Science and Clinical Applications. New York, Pergamon Press, 1989, S. 139–155

Arnoult JB, Vila-Coro AA, Mazow ML. Goniotomy with sodium hyaluronate. J Pediatric Ophthalmology 25:18–22

Aron-Rosa D, Cohn HC, Aron J-J, Boquety C. Methylcellulose instead of Healon® in extracapsular surgery with intraocular lens implantation. Ophthalmology 1983; 90:1235–1238

Arshinoff SA. Viscoelastic substances: their properties and use when placing an IOL in the capsular bag. Curr Can Ophthalmic Prac 1986; 4:64–65; 72; 74

Arshinoff SA. Comparative physical properties of ophthalmic viscoelastic materials. Curr Can Ophthalmic Prac 1989; 7:1

Arshinoff SA. The physical properties of ophthalmic viscoelastics in cataract surgery. Ophthalmic Pract 1991; 9:81–86

Arshinoff SA. Mechanics of capsulorhexis. J Cataract Refract Surg 1992; 18:623–628

Arshinoff SA. Dispersive and cohesive viscoelastic materials in phacoemulsification. Ophthalmic Pract 1995; 13:98–104

Arshinoff SA, Hofmann I. Prospective, randomized trial of Microvisc® and Healon® in routine phacoemulsification. J Cataract Refract Surg 1997; 23:761–765

Arshinoff SA. Dispersive and cohesive viscoelastic materials in phacoemulsification revisited 1998. Ophthalmic Practice 1998; 16:24–32

Arshinoff SA. Dispersive-cohesive viscoelastic soft shell technique. J Cataract Refract Surg 1999; 25:167-173

Artola A, Alió JL, Bellot JL, Ruiz JM. Lipid peroxidation in the iris and its protection by means of viscoelastic substances (Sodium hyaluronate and hydroxypropylmethylcellulose). Ophthalmic Res 1993; 25:172–176

Arzeno A, Miller D. Effect of sodium hyaluronate on corneal wound healing. Arch Ophthalmol 1982; 100:152

Assia EI, Apple DJ, Lim ES, Morgan RC, Tsai JC. Removal of viscoelastic material after experimental cataract surgery in vitro. J Cataract Refract Surg 1992; 18:3–6

Auffarth GU, Wesendahl TA, Solomon KD, Brown SJ, Apple DJ. Evaluation of different removal techniques of a high-viscosity viscoelastic. J Cataract Refract Surg 1994; best papers of session

Baba T, Kasahara A, Momose A. Use of methylcellulose in cataract extraction and IOL implantation. Proceedings of the XXV International Congress of Ophthalmology. Rome, 1986. Amsterdam, Kugler and Ghedini, 1987, S. 1004–1006

Balazs EA. Physiology of the vitreous body. Schepens CL (ed): Importance of the vitreous body in retina surgery with special emphasis on reoperations. St. Louis, C.V. Mosby, 1960, S. 29–48

Balazs EA, Gibbs DA. The rheological properties and biological function of hyaluronic acid, in Balazs EA (ed). Chemistry and Molecular Biology of the Intercellular Matrix, Vol 3. London, Academic Press, 1970, S. 1241–1253

Balazs EA, Freeman MI, Klöti R, Meyer-Schwickerath O, Regnault F, Sweeney DH. Hyaluronic acid and the replacement of vitreous and aqueous humor. Mod Probl Ophthalmol 1972; 10:3–21

Balazs EA, Darzynkiewisz Z. The effect of hyaluronic acid on fibroblasts, mononuclear phagocytes and lymphocytes. In: E. Kulonen, J. Pikkarainen (eds.): Biology of the fibroblast. London, Academic Press, 1973, S. 237–252

Balazs EA, Hutsch E. Replacement of the vitreous with hyaluronic acid, collagen and other polymers. Irvine AR, O'Malley C (eds): Advances in Vitreous Surgery. Springfield, Illinois, Charles C Thomas, 1976, S. 601–623

Balazs EA. Ultrapure hyaluronic acid and the use thereof. US Patent No. 4.141.973, Oct. 17, 1979

Balazs EA. Sodium hyaluronate and viscosurgery. Miller D, Stegmann R (eds): Healon®, A Guide to Its Use in Ophthalmic Surgery. New York, Wiley Medical Publishers, 1983, S. 5–28

Balazs EA. Pharmakologische Eigenschaften von Natrium-Hyaluronat im Auge. In: Meyer-Schwickerath G (Hrsg) Viskochirurgie des Auges. Enke, Stuttgart, 1984; S. 1–13

Balazs EA. Viscosurgery, features of a true viscosurgical tool and its role in ophthalmic surgery, in Miller D, Stegmann R (eds): Treatment of Anterior Segment Ocular Trauma. Montreal, Canada, Medicöpea, 1986a, S. 121–128

Balazs EA, Freeman MI, Regnault F. The development of sodium hyaluronate (Healon®) as a viscoelastic material in ophthalmic surgery, in Eisner G (ed): Ophthalmic Viscosurgery: A Review of Standards, Techniques and Applications. Bern, Switzerland, Medicopea International, 1986b, S. 3–19

Balazs EA. The introduction of elastoviscous hyaluron for viscosurgery. Rosen ES (ed): Viscoelastic Materials: Basic Science and Clinical Applications. New York, Pergamon Press, 1989, S. 167–183

Baldwin LB, Smith TJ, Holkins JL, Pearson PA. The use of viscoelastic substances in the drainage of postoperative suprachoroidal hemorrhage. Ophthalmic Surg 1989; 20:504–507

Barak A, Alhalel A, Kotas R, Melamed S. The protective effect of early intraoperative injection of viscoelastic material in trabeculectomy. Ophthalmic Surg 1992; 23:206–209

Barak A, Desatnik H, Ma-Naim T, Ashkenasi I, Neufeld A, Melamed S. Early postoperative intraocular pressure pattern in glaucomatous and nonglaucomatous patients. J Cataract Refract Surg 1996; 22:607–611

Bárány EH. The action of different kinds of hyaluronidase on the resistance to flow through the angle of the anterior chamber. Acta Ophthalmol (Copenh) 1956; 34:397–403

Barron BA, Busin M, Page C, Bergsma DR, Kaufman HE. Comparison of the effects of Viscoat and Healon on postoperative intraocular pressure. Am J Ophthalmol 1985; 100: 377–384

Bartholomew RS. Viscoelastic evacuation of traumatic hyphaema. Br J Ophthalmol 1987; 71:27–28

Baotis S, Nayak H, Mathur U. Capsular bag distension after optic capture of a sulans-fixated intraocular lens. J Cataract Refract Surg 1999; 25:293-295

Becker KW, Ehrich W, Höh H. Hornhauttrübungen und Irisfältchen beim Vorderkammer-implantationstest am Kaninchenauge – Spaltlampenmikroskopische und histologische Befunde. Contactologica 1988; 10:115-121

Berson FG, Patterson MM, Epstein DL. Obstruction of aqueous outflow by sodium hyaluronate in enculeated human eyes. Am J Ophthalmol 1983; 95:668–672

Bigar F, Gloor B, Schimmelpfennig B, Thumm D. Die Verträglichkeit von Hydroxypropylmethylcellulose bei der Implantation von Hinterkammerlinsen. Klin Monatsbl Augenheilkd 1988; 193:21–24

Binder PS, Deg JK, Kohl FS. Calcific band keratopathy after intraocular chondroitin sulfate. Arch Ophthalmol 1987; 105:1243–1247

Bleckmann H, Vogt R, Garus H-J. Collagel – a new viscoelastic substance for ophthalmic surgery. J Cataract Refract Surg 1992; 18:20–26

Blondeau P. Sodium hyaluronate in trabeculectomy: A retrospective study. Can J Ophthalmol 1984; 19:306–309

Bothner H, Wik O. Rheology of hyaluronate. Acta Otolaryngol (Stockh) 1987; 442(Suppl):25–30

Bothner H, Wik O. Rheology of intraocular solutions. Rosen ES (ed): Viscoelastic Materials: Basic Science and Clinical Applications. New York, Pergamon Press, 1989, S. 3–22

Bourne WM, Brubaker RF, O'Fallon WM. Use of air to decrease endothelial cell loss during intraocular lens implantation. Arch Ophthalmol 1979; 97:1473–1475

Bourne WM, Liesegang TJ, Waller RR, Ilstrup DM. The effect of sodium hyaluronate on endothelial cell damage during extracapsular cataract extraction and posterior chamber lens implantation. Am J Ophthalmol 1984, 98:759–762

Brauweiler P. Bimanual irrigation/aspiration. J Cataract Refract Surg 1996; 22:1013–1016

Bresciani C, Lebuisson DA, Eveillard M, Grossiord JL, Drupt F, Montefiore G. Dynamic viscosity and corneal endothelial protection with Healonid, Healon GV, Provisc and Viscoat during phacoemulsification. J Fr Ophthalmol 1996; 19:39–50

Brown GC, Benson WE. Use of sodium hyaluronate for the repair of giant retinal tears. Arch Ophthalmol 1989; 107:1246–1249

Buckley RJ. Healthy corneal endothelium and the effects of intraocular surgery. Trans Ophthalmol Soc UK 1985; 104:801–826

Burke S, Sugar J, Farber MD. Comparison of the effects of two viscoelastic agents, Healon and Viscoat, on postoperative intraocular pressure after penetrating keratoplasty. Ophthalmic Surg 1990; 21:821–826

Buschmann DM. Numerical conversion of transient to harmonic response functions for linear viscoelastic materials. J Biomechanics 1997; 30:197–202

Cadera W, Harding PW, Gonder JR, Hooper PL. Management of severe hypotony with intravitreal injection of Healon. Can J Ophthalmol 1993; 28:236–237

Cairns JE. Trabeculectomy. Am J Ophthalmol 1968; 66:673–679

Calder IG, Smith VH. Hyaluronidase and sodium hyaluronate in cataract surgery. Br J Ophthalmol 1986, 70:418–420

Campbell DG, Vela A. Modern goniosynechialysis for the treatment of synechial angle-closure glaucoma. Ophthalmology 1984; 91:1052–1060

Charlier J-P, Crowet F. Wave equations in linear viscoelastic materials. J Acoust Soc Am 1986; 79:895–900

Charleux J, Dupont D, Charleux M, et al. Human placental collagen type IV: An alternative as viscoplastic solution in ocular microsurgery. Proceedings of the XXV International Congress of Ophthalmology. Rome 1986. Amsterdam, Kugler and Ghedini, 1987, S. 1066–1067

Charleux J, Charleux M, Dupont D, et al. Le collagène IV visqueux d'origine humaine; propriétés physiques et tolérance expérimentale. Ophthalmologie 1989; 3:308–311

Charteris DG, McConell JMS, Adams AD. Effect of sodium hyaluronate on trabeculectomy filtration blebs. J R Coll Surg Eding 1991; 36:107–108

Cherfan GM, Rich WJ, Wright G. Raised intraocular pressure and other problems with sodium hyaluronate and cataract surgery. Trans Ophthalmol Soc UK 1983; 103:277–279

Chung J-H, Kim H-J, Fagerholm P, Cho B-C. Effect of topically applied Na-hyaluronan on experimental corneal alkali wound healing. Korean J Ophthalmol 1996; 10:68–75

Clorfeine GS, Parker WT. Use of Healon in eye muscle surgery with adjustable sutures. Ann Ophthalmol 1987; 19:215–217

Coffman MR, Mann PM. Corneal subepithelial deposits after use of sodium chondroitin. Am J Ophthalmol 1986; 102:279–280

Colin J, Durand L, Mouillon M, Lagoutte F, Constantinides G, Villard C, Romanet J-P. Comparative clinical trial of AMO Vitrax and Healon use in extracapsular cataract extraction. J Cataract Refract Surg 1995; 21:196–201

Comper WD, Laurent TC. Physiological function of connective tissue polysaccharides. Physiol Rev 1978; 58:255–315

Condon PI, Fitzgerald G, Burke A, Gallagher J. The physical effects of viscoelastic substances on human donor cornea. Trans Ophthalmol Soc UK 1983; 103:265–267

Condon PJ, Gillan J, Mullaney J, Hurley M, Kinsella M. Ultrastuctural studies of the effect of viscoelastic substances on the endothelium of human donor corneae – a pilot study. In: Rosen ES (ed): Viscoelastic Materials: Basic Science and Clinical Applications. New York, Pergamon Press 1989, S. 91–100

Crafoord S, Stenkula S. Healon® GV in posterior segment surgery. Acta Ophthalmologica 1993; 71:560–561

Craig MT, Olson RJ, Mamalis N, Olson RJ. Air bubble endothelial damage during phacoemulsification in human eye bank eyes: The protective effects of Healon® and Viscoat®. J Cataract Refract Surg 1990; 16:597–602

Daniele S, Refojo MF, Schepens CL, Freeman HM. Gylceryl methacrylate hydrogel as a vitreous implant. Arch Ophthalmol 1968; 80:120–127

Darzynkiewisz Z, Balazs EA. Effect of connective tissue intercellular matrix on lymphocyte stimulation. I. Suppression of lymphocyte stimulation by hyaluronic acid. Exp Cell Res 1971; 66:113–123

Davison JA. Capsular bag distension after endophacoemulsification and posterior chamber intraocular lens implantation. J Cataract Refract Surg 190; 16:99-108

DeLuise VP, Peterson WJ. The use of topical Healon tears in the management of refractory dry-eye syndrome. Ann Ophthalmol 1984; 16:823–824

Denffer H v, Fabian E. Healon® in der Versorgung perforierender Augenverletzungen. In: Meyer-Schwickerath G (Hrsg) Viskochirurgie des Auges. Enke, Stuttgart, 1984; S. 81–87

Denlinger JL, Balazs EA. Replacement of the liquid vitreous with sodium hyaluronate in monkeys. I. Short-term evaluation. Exp Eye Res 1980a; 31:81–99

Denlinger JL, Schubert H, Balazs EA. Na hyaluronate of various molecular sizes injected into the anterior chamber of owl monkey: disappearance and effect on intraocular pressure. Proc Int Soc Eye Res 1980b; 1:88

Denlinger JL, Balazs EA. The fate of exogenous viscoelastic hyaluronan solutions in the primate eye. Rosen ES (ed): Viscoelastic Materials: Basic Science and Clinical Applications. New York, Pergamon Press, 1989, S. 185–199

D'Ermo F, Bonomi L, Duro D. A critical analysis of the long-term results of trabeculectomy. Am J Ophthalmol 1979; 88:829–835

Dick HB, Kohnen T, Jacobi FK, Jacobi KW. Long-term endothelial cell loss following phacoemulsification through temporal clear corneal incision. J Cataract Refract Surg 1996; 22:63–71

Dick HB, Schwenn O, Pfeiffer N. Einteilung der viskoelastischen Substanzen für die Ophthalmochirurgie. Ophthalmologe 1999; 96:193-211

Dick HB, Schwenn O, Fabian E, Neuhann T, Eisenmann D. Cartridge cracks with different viscoelastic agents (letter). J Cataract Refract Surg 1999; 25:463-465

Dick HB, Krummenauer F, Vogel A, Pakula T, Pfeiffer N. Healon®5: a viscoadaptive formulation compared to Healon® and Healon® GV. J Cataract Refract Surg 2000; (in press)

Draeger J, Winter R, Wirth H. Viscoelastic glaucoma surgery. Trans Ophthalmol Soc UK 1983; 103:270–273

Drews RC. Sodium hyaluronate (Healon®) in the repair of perforating injuries of the eye. Ophthalmic Surg 1986; 17:23–29

Drews RC, Gabrawy L. Blue Healon®. J Cataract Refract Surg 1989; 15:100–104

Dunn M, Stenzel KH, Rubin AL, Miyata T. Collagen implants in the vitreous. Arch Ophthalmol 1969; 82:840–844

Duperre J, Grenier B, Lemire J, Mihalovits H, Sebag M, Lambert J. Effect of timolol vs. acetazolamide on sodium hyaluronate-induced rise in intraocular pressure after cataract surgery. Can J Ophthalmol 1994; 29:182–186

Eason J, Seward HC. Pupil size and reactivity following hydroxypropyl methylcellulose and sodium hyaluronate. Br J Ophthalmol 1995; 79:541–543

Edelhauser HF, Hanneken AM, Pederson HJ, van Horn DL. Osmotic tolerance of rabbit and human corneal endothelium. Arch Ophthalmol 1981; 99:1281–1287

Edelhauser HF, MacRae SM. Irrigating and viscous solutions. In: Sears M, Tarkkanen A (eds) Surgical Pharmacology of the Eye. New York, Raven Press, 1985

Ehrich W. Vorderkammertest von Kunststoffen für Kontaktlinsen und Intraokluarlinsen. Contactologica 1987; 4:1–2

Ehrich W, Höh H, Kreiner CF. Biologische Verträglichkeit und Pharmakokinetik von Hydroxypropyl-methylcellulose (HPMC) in der Vorderkammer des Kaninchenauges. Klin Monatsbl Augenheilkd 1990; 196:470–474

Eiferman RA, Wilkins EL. The effect of air on human corneal endothelium. Am J Ophthalmol 1981; 92:328–331

Eisner G. Eye Surgery. An Introduction to Operative Technique. New York, Springer Berlin Heidelberg New York Tokio, 1980, S. 171–181

Eisner G. Der raumtaktische Einsatz einer viskösen Substanz (Healon®). Klin Monatsbl Augenheilkd 1981; 178:32–39

Eisner G. General considerations concerning viscous materials in ophthalmic surgery. Trans Ophthal Soc UK 1983; 103:247–253

Embriano PJ. Postoperative pressure after phacoemulsification: sodium hyaluronate vs. sodium chondroitin sulfate – sodium hyaluronate. Ann Ophthalmol 1989; 21:85–90

Fechner PU. Methylcellulose in lens implantation. J Am Intraocul Soc 1977; 3:180–181

Fechner PU, Fechner MU. Methylcellulose and lens implantation. Br J Ophthalmol 1983; 67:259–263

Fechner PU. Preparation of 2% hydroxypropyl methylcellulose for viscous surgery. J Am Intraocul Implant Soc 1985; 11:606–607

Federman J, Decker WL, Grabowski WM. Cover slip lens. Am J Ophthalmol 1983; 95:848–849

Fernandez-Vigo J, Refojo MF, Jumblatt M. Elimination of hydroxypropyl methylcellulose from the anterior chamber of the rabbit. J Cataract Refract Surg 1989; 15:191–195

Ferreira RC, Lamberts M, Moreira JB, Campos MS. Hydroxypropylmethylcellulose and sodium hyaluronate in adjustable strabismus surgery. J Pediatr Ophthalmol Strabismus 1995; 32:239–242

Fine IH, Hoffman RS. Late reopening of fibrosed capsular bags to reposition decentered intraocular lenses. J Cataract Refract Surg 1997; 23:990–994

Fisher YL, Turtz AI, Gold M. Use of sodium hyaluronate in reformation and reconstruction of the persistent flat anterior chamber in the presence of severe hypotony. Ophthalmic Surg 1982; 13: 819–821

Florén I, Hansen R, Ehinger B. Endophthalmitis-like reaction to viscoelastic material. XVth Congress of the European Society of Cataract 24:145–146

Folk JC, Packer AJ, Weingeist TA, Howcraft MJ. Sodium hyaluronate (Healon®) in closed vitrectomy. Ophthalmic Surg 1986; 17:299–306

Forrester JV, Wilkinson PC. Inhibition of leikocyte locomotion by hyaluronic acid. J Cell Sci 1981; 48:315–331

Forsberg N, Von Malmborg A, Madsen K, Rolfsen W, Gustafson S. Receptors for hyaluronan on corneal endothelial cells. Exp Eye Res 1994; 59:689–696

Fourman S. Management of cornea-lens touch after filtering surgery for glaucoma. Ophthalmol 1990; 97:424–428

Fraser JRE, Laurent TC, Pertoft H, Baxter E. Plasma clearance, tissue distribution and metabolism of hyaluronic acid injected intravenously in the rabbit. Biochem J 1981; 200:415–424

Friedburg D. Visco-hydraulic irrigation of the lens cortex. A safe ECCE method. Klin Monatsbl Augenheilkd 1994; 205:344–347

Frohn A, Dick HB, Fritzen CP, Breitenbach M, Thiel HJ. Ultrasonic transmission in viscoelastic substances. J Cataract Refract Surg 2000; 26:282–286

Fry LL. Postoperative intraocular pressure rises: A comparison of Healon, Amvisc, and Viscoat. J Cataract Refract Surg 1989; 15:415–420

Fry LL. Comparison of the postoperative intraocular pressure with Betagan, Betoptic, Timoptic, Iopidine, Diamox, Pilopine Gel, and Miostat. J Cataract Refract Surg 1992; 18:14–19

Fry LL, Yee RW. Healon GV in extracapsular cataract extraction with intraocular lens implantation. J Cataract Refract Surg 1993; 19:409–412

Gandolfi SA, Massari A, Orsoni JG. Low-molecular-weight sodium hyaluronate in the treatment of bacterial corneal ulcers. Graefe's Arch Clin Exp Ophthalmol 1992; 230:20–23

Gaskell A, Haining WM. A double blind randomized multicentre clinical trial of „Healon G.V." compared with „Healon" in ECCE with IOL implantation. Eur J Implant Refract Surg 1991; 3:241–244

Gerke E, Meyer-Schwickerath G, Siebert A. Healon® bei Netzhautablösung. In: Meyer-Schwickerath G (Hrsg) Viskochirurgie des Auges. Enke, Stuttgart, 1984; S. 99–103

Gibbs DA, Merrill EW, Smith KA, Balazs EA. Rheology of hyaluronic acid. Bipolymers 1968; 6:777–791

Gimbel HV, Ferensowicz M, Raanan M, DeLuca M. Implantation in children. J Pediatr Ophthalmol Strabismus 1993; 30:69–79

Glasser DB, Matsuda M, Ellis JG, Edelhauser HF. Effects of intraocular solutions on the corneal endothelium after in vivo anterior chamber irrigation. Am J Ophthalmol 1985; 99:321–328

Glasser DB, Matsuda M, Edelhauser HF. A comparison of the efficacy and toxicity of and intraocular pressure response to viscous solutions in the anterior chamber. Arch Ophthalmol 1986; 104:1819–1824

Glasser DB, Katz HR, Boyd JE, Langdon JD, Shobe SL, Peiffer RL. Protective effects of viscous solutions in phacoemulsification and traumatic lens implantation. Arch Ophthalmol 1989; 107:1047–1051

Glasser DB, Osborn DC, Nordeen JF, Min Y. Endothelial protection and viscoelastic retention during phacoemulsification and intraocular lens implantation. Arch Ophthalmol 1991; 109:1438–1440

Gombos GM, Berman ER. Chemical and clinical observations on the fate of various vitreous substitutes. Acta Ophthalmol 1967; 45:794–805

Gonnering R, Edelhauser HF, van Horn DL, Durant W. The pH tolerance of rabbit and human corneal endothelium. Invest Ophthalmol Vis Sci 1979; 18:373–390

Graue EL, Polack FM, Balazs EA. The protective effect of Na-hyaluronate to corneal endothelium. Exp Eye Res 1980; 31:119–127

Grisanti S, Jacobi PC, Bartz-Schmidt KU, Heimann K. Pseudoendophthalmitis after the use of a new viscoelastic product. XVth Congress of the European Society of Cataract 105:466–469

Gruber PF, Schipper I, Kem R. Use of Healon for corneal trephination in penetrating keratoplasty. Ophthalmic Surg 1984; 15:773

Guthoff R, Wendl U, Böhnke M, Winter R. Endothelzellschützende Wirkung hochviskÖser Substanzen in der Kataraktchirurgie. Ophthalmologe 1992; 89:310–312

Härfstrand A, Molander N, Stenevi U, Apple D, Schenholm M, Madsen K. Evidence of hyaluronic acid and hyaluronic acid binding sites on human corneal endothelium. J Cataract Refract Surg 1992; 18:265–269

Hamano T, Horimoto K, Lee M, Komemushi S. Sodium hyaluronate eyedrops enhance tear film stability. Jpn J Ophthalmol 1996; 40:62–65

Hammer ME, Burch TG. Viscous corneal protection by sodium hyaluronate, chondroitin sulfate, and methylcellulose. Invest Ophthalmol Vis Sci 1984; 25:1329–1332

Harrison SE, Soll DB, Shayegan M. Clinch T. Chondroitin sulfate: a new and effective protective agent for intraocular lens insertion. Ophthalmology 1982; 89:1254–1260

Hayreh SS. Anterior ischemic optic neuropathy. Occurrence after cataract extraction. Arch Ophthalmol 1980; 98:1410–1416

Hedbys BO. The role of polysaccharide in corneal swelling. Exp Eye Res 1963; 2:122–129

Hein SR; Keates RH, Weber PA. Elimination of sodium hyaluronate-induced decrease in outflow facility with hyaluronidase. Ophthalmic Surg 1986; 17:731–734

Henry JC, Olander K. Comparison of the effect of four viscoelastic agents on early postoperative intraocular pressure. J Cataract Refract Surg 1996; 22:960–966

Herrington RG, Ball SF, Updegraff SA. Delayed sustained increase in intraocular pressure secondary to the use of polyacrylamide gel (Orcolon®) in the anterior chamber. Ophthalmic Surg 1993; 24:658–662

Hessemer V, Dick B. Viskoelastische Substanzen in der Kataraktchirurgie – Grundlagen und aktuelle Übersicht. Klin Monatsbl Augenheilkd 1996; 208:55–61

Hirst LW, DeJuan E Jr. Sodium hyaluronate and tissue adhesive in treating corneal perforations. Ophthalmology 1982; 89:1250–1253

Hoffer KJ. Effects of extracapsular implant techniques on endothelial density. Arch Ophthalmol 1982; 100:791–792

Holmberg ÅS, Philipson BT. Sodium hyaluronate in cataract surgery. I. Report on the use of Healon® in two different types of intracapsular cataract surgery. Ophthalmology 1984a; 91:45–52

Holmberg ÅS, Philipson BT. Sodium hyaluronate in cataract surgery. II. Report on the use of Healon® in extracapsular cataract surgery using phacoemulsification. Ophthalmology 1984b; 91:53–59

Holst A, Rolfsen W, Svensson B, Öllinger K, Lundgren B. Formation of free radicals during phacoemulsification. Curr Eye Res 1993; 12:359–365

Hütz WW, Eckhardt B, Kohnen T. Comparison of viscoelastic substances used in phacoemulsification. J Cataract Refract Surg 1996; 22:955–959

Hultsch E. The scope of hyaluronic acid as an experimental intraocular implant. Ophthalmology 1980; 87:706–712

Hung SO. Role of sodium hyaluronate (Healonid) in triangular flap trabeculectomy. Br J Ophthalmol 1985; 69:46–50

Hyndiuk RA, Schultz RO. Overview of the corneal toxicity of surgical solutions and drugs and clinical concepts in corneal edema. Lens Eye Toxic Res 1992; 9:331–350

Imkamp E, Kaden P, Kuss M, Hunold W, Mittermayer C. Konzentrationsabhängige Effekte viskochirurgischer Substanzen auf das Zellwachstum boviner Kornea-Endothelzellen. Fortschr Ophthalmol 1988; 85:434–436

Insler MS. A new use for sodium hyaluronate (Healon) in penetrating keratoplasty. Ann Ophthalmol 1985; 17:106–107

Iwata S, Miyauchi S, Takehana M. Biochemical studies on the use of sodium hyaluronate in the anterior eye segment. I. Variation of protein and ascorbic acid concentration in rabbit aqueous humor. Curr Eye Res 1984; 3:605–610

Iwata S, Miyauchi S. Biochemical studies on the use of sodium hyaluronate in the anterior eye segment. III. Histological studies on distribution and efflux process of 5-Aminofluorescein-labeled hyaluronate. Jpn J Ophthalmol 1985; 29:187–197

Jensen MK, Crandall AS, Mamalis N, Olson RJ. Crystallization on intraocular lens surfaces associated with the use of Healon GV. Arch Ophthalmol 1994; 112:1037–1042

Juzych MS, Parras KA, Shin DH, Swebdris RP, Ramocki JM. Adjunctive viscoelastic therapy for postoperative ciliary block. Ophthalmic Surg 1992; 23:784–788

Kammann J, Dornbach G, Vollenberg C, Hille P. Kontrollierte klinische Studie zweier viskoelastischer Substanzen. Fortschr Ophthalmol 1991; 88:438–441

Kanellopoulos AJ, Perry HD, Donnenfeld ED. Timolol gel versus acetazolamide in the prophylaxis of ocular hypertension after phacoemulsification. J Cataract Refract Surg 1997a; 23:1070–1074

Kanellopoulos AJ, Perry HD, Donnenfeld ED. Comparison of topical timolol gel to oral acetazolamid in the prophylaxis of viscoelastic-induced ocular hypertension after penetrating keratoplasty. Cornea 1997b; 16:12–15

Karel I, Kalvodova B, Filipec M, Bohacova E, Soucek P, Povysil C, Vacik J, Tlustakova M. Poly(triethylenglycol monomethacrylate) and poly(glycerol monomethacrylate) cross-linked gel as potential viscoelastics for intraoperative use. Graefe's Archive Clin Exp Ophthalmol 1997; 235:186–189

Kassar BS, Varnell ED. Effect of PMMA and silicone lens materials on normal rabbit corneal endothelium: An in vitro study. Am Intra-Ocular Implant Soc J 1982; 8:55–58

Kaufman PL, Lütjen-Dcroll E, Hubbard BS, Erikson KA. Obstruction of aqueous humor outflow by cross-linked polyacrylamid microgels in bovine, monkey and human eyes. Ophthalmology 1994; 101:1672–1679

Keates RH, Powell J, Blosser E. Coated intraocular lenses. Ophthalmic Surg 1987; 18:693–697

Kelman CD. Rhaco-emulsification and aspiration. A new technique of cataract removal. A preliminary report. Am J Ophthalmol 1967; 64:23–25

Kerr Muir MG, Sherrard ES, Andrews V, Steel ADM. Air, methylcellulose, sodium hyaluronate and the corneal endothelium: endothelial protective agents. Eye 1987; 1:480–486

Kim JH. Intraocular inflammation of denatured viscoelastic substance in cases of cataract extraction and lens implantation. J Cataract Refract Surg 1987; 13:537–542

Kirkby GR, Gregor ZJ. The removal of silicone oil from the anterior chamber in phakic eyes. Arch Ophthalmol 1987; 105:1592

Kishimoto M, Yamanouchi U, Mori F, Nakamori F. An experimental study on the substitute of the vitreous body. Acta Soc Ophthalmol Jap 1964; 68:1145

Klemm M, Balazs A, Draeger J, Wiezorrek R. Experimental use of space-retaining substances with extended duration: functional and morphological results. Graefe's Arch Clin Exp Ophthalmol 1995; 233:592–597

Koch DD, Liu JF, Glasser DB, Merin LM, Haft E. A comparison of corneal endothelial changes after use of Healon® or Viscoat® during phacoemulsification. Am J Ophthalmol 1993; 115:188–201

Kohnen T, von Ehr M, Schütte E. Postoperativer Druckverlauf in den ersten Tagen nach intraokularem Einsatz von Hyaluronsäurelösung mit unterschiedlicher Viskosität. Klin Monatsbl Augenheilkd 1995; 207:29–36

Kohnen T, von Ehr M, Schütte E, Koch DD. Evaluation of intraocular pressure with Healon® and Healon® GV in sutureless cataract surgery with foldable lens implantation. J Cataract Refract Surg 1996; 22:227–237

Koster R, Stilma JS. Comparison of vitreous replacement with Healon® and with HPMC in rabbits' eyes. Doc Ophthalmol 1986a; 61:247–253

Koster R, Stilma JS. Healon® as intravitreal substitute in retinal-detachment surgery in 40 patients. Doc Ophthalmol 1986b; 64:13–17

Kwitko S, Belfort R Jr. Light and electron microscopic analysis of intraocular 2% hydroxypropylmethylcellulose. J Cataract Refract Surg 1991; 17:478–484

Landers MB III. Sodium hyaluronate (Healon) as an aid to internal fluid-gas exchange (letter to the editor). Am J Ophthalmol 1982; 94:557–558

Lane SS, Naylor DW, Kullerstrand LJ, Knauth K, Lindstrom RL. Prospective comparison of the effects of Ocucoat®, Viscoat®, and Healon® on intraocular pressure and endothelial cell loss. J Cataract Refract Surg 1991; 17:21–26

Lang E, Mark D, Miller FA, Miller D, Wik O. Shear flow characteristics of sodium hyaluronate: relationship to performance in anterior segment surgery. Arch Ophthalmol 1984; 102:1079–1082

Laurell C-G, Philipson B. An open randomized clinical study comparing Healon® GV and Healon® during soft IOL implantation. Eur J Impl Ref Surg 1995; 7:170–172

Laurent TC. A comparative study of physico-chemical properties of hyaluronic acid prepared according to different methods and from different tissues. Ark Kemi 1957; 11:487–496

Laurent UBG, Laurent TC. On the origin of hyaluronate in blood. Biochem Int 1981; 2:195–199

Laurent UBG, Granath KA. The molecular weight of hyaluronate in the aqueous humour and vitreous body of rabbit and cattle eyes. Exp Eye Res 1983; 36:481–492

Laurent UBG, Fraser JRE. Disappearance of concentrated hyaluronan from the anterior chamber of monkey eyes. Exp Eye Res 1990; 51:65–69

Laurent UBG, Dahl LB, Lilja K. Hyaluronan injected in the anterior chamber of the eye is catabolized in the liver. Exp Eye Res 1993; 57:435–440

Leaming DV. Practice styles and preferences of ASCRS members – 1990 survey. J Cataract Refract Surg 1991; 17:495–502

Leaming DV. Practice styles and preferences of ASCRS members – 1991 survey. J Cataract Refract Surg 1992; 18:460–469

Leaming DV. Practice styles and preferences of ASCRS members – 1992 survey. J Cataract Refract Surg 1993; 19:600–606

Leaming DV. Practice styles and preferences of ASCRS members – 1993 survey. J Cataract Refract Surg 1994; 20:459–467

Leaming DV. Practice styles and preferences of ASCRS members – 1994 survey. J Cataract Refract Surg 1995; 21:378–385

Leaming DV. Practice styles and preferences of ASCRS members – 1995 survey. J Cataract Refract Surg 1996; 22:931–939

Leaming DV. Practice styles and preferences of ASCRS members – 1996 survey. J Cataract Refract Surg 1997; 23:527–535

Leaming DV. Practice styles and preferences of ASCRS members – 1997 survey. J Cataract Refract Surg 1998; 24:552–561

Leaming DV. Practice styles and preferences of ASCRS members – 1998 survey. J Cataract Refract Surg 1999; 25:851–859

Lehmann R, Brint S, Stewart R, White GL Jr, McCarthy G, Taylor R, Disbrow D, Defaller J. Clinical comparison of Provisc and Healon in cataract surgery. J Cataract Refract Surg 1995; 20:543–547

Leith MM, Loftus SA, Kuo J-W, DeVore DP, Keates EU. Comparison of the properties of AMVISC® and Healon®. J Cataract Refract Surg 1987; 13:534–536

Lemp MA. The use of sodium hyaluronate (Healon) in the removal of corneal foreign body with a perforating corneal laceration. Cornea 1982; 1:357–358

Lerner HA, Boynton JR. Sodium hyaluronate (Healon®) as an adjunct to lacrimal surgery (letter to the editor). Am J Ophthalmol 1985; 99:365

Levy NS, Boone L. Effect of hyaluronic acid viscosity on IOP elevation after cataract surgery. Glaucoma 1989; 11:82–85

Lewen R, Insler MS. The effect of prophylactic acetazolamide on the intraocular pressure rise associated with Healon-aided intraocular lens surgery. Ann Ophthalmol 1985; 17:315–318

Lewis JM, Ohji M, Tano Y. The use of sodium hyaluronate to view the fundus during vitreous surgery. Retina 1996; 16:447–449

Liesegang TJ, Bourne WM, Ilstrup DM. The use of hydroxypropyl methylcellulose in extracapsular cataract extraction with intraocular lens implantation. Am J Ophthalmol 1986; 102:723–726

Liesegang TJ. Viscoelastic substances in ophthalmology. Surv Ophthalmol 1990; 34:268–293

Limberg MB, McCaa C, Kissling GE, Kaufman HE. Topical application of hyaluronic acid and chondroitin sulfate in the treatment of dry eyes. Am J Ophthalmol 1987; 103:194–197

Lindquist TD, Edenfield M. Cytotoxicity of viscoelastics on cultured corneal epithelial cells measured by plasminogen activator release. J Refract Corneal Surg 1994; 10:95–102

MacRae SM, Edelhauser HF, Hyndiuk RA, Burd EM, Schultz RO. The effects of sodium hyaluronate, chondroitin sulfate, and methylcellulose on the corneal endothelium and intraocular pressure. Am J Ophthalmol 1983; 95:332–341

Madsen K, Stenevi U, Aplle DJ, Härfstrand A. Histochemical and receptor binding studies of hyaluronic acid and hyaluronic acid binding sites on corneal endothelium. Ophthalmic Practice 1989a; 7:92–97

Madsen K, Schenholm M, Jahnke G, Tengblad A. Hyaluronate binding to intact corneas and cultured endothelial cells. Invest Ophthalmol Vis Sci 1989b; 30:2132–2137

Maguen E, Nesburn AB, Macy JI. Combined use of sodium hyaluronate and tissue adhesive in penetrating keratoplasty of corneal perforations. Ophthalmic Surg 1984; 15:55–57

Mandelcorn M. Viscoelastic dissection for relocation of off-axis intraocular lens implant: a new technique. Can J Ophthalmol 1995; 30:34–35

McAuliffe KM. Sodium hyaluronate in the treatment of Descemet's membrane detachment. J Ocul Ther Surg 1982; 1:58–59

McDermott ML, Edelhauser HF. Drug binding of ophthalmic viscoelastic agents. Arch Ophthalmol 1989; 107:261–263

McDermott ML, Hazlett LD, Barrett RP, Lambert RJ. Viscoelastic adherence to corneal endothelium following phacoemulsification. J Cataract Refract Surg 1998; 24:678–683

McKnight SJ, Giangiacomo J, Adelstein E. Inflammatory response to viscoelastic materials. Ophthalmic Surg 1987; 18:804–806

McLeod D. James CR. Viscodelaminiation at the vitreoretinal juncture in severe diabetic eye disease. Br J Ophthalmol 1988; 72:413–419

Meaney DF. Mechanical properties of implantable biomaterials. Clinics in podiatric medicine and surgery 1995; 12:363–384

Medizinproduktegesetz vom 2. August 1994

Melles GR, Lander F, Rietfield FJ, Remeijer L, Beekhuis WH, Binder PS. A new surgical technique for deep stromae, anterior lamellar keratoplasty. Br J Ophthalmol 1999; 83:327-333

Menezo JL, Taboada JF, Ferrer E. Complications of intraocular lenses in children. Trans Ophthalmol Soc UK 1985; 104:546–552

Mengher LS, Pandher KS, Bron AJ, Davey CC. Effect of sodium hyaluronate (0.1%) on break-up time (NIBUT) in patients with dry eyes. Br J Ophthalmol 1986; 70:442–447

Meyer DR, McCulley JP. Different prospects of risk management from in vitro toxicology and its relevance to the evolution of viscoelastic formulations. Rosen ES (ed): Viscoelastic Materials: Basic Science and Clinical Applications. New York, Pergamon Press, 1989, S. 45–90

Meyer K, Palmer JW. The polysaccharide of the vitreous humor. J Biol Chem 1934; 107:629–634

Meyer K. Chemical structure of hyaluronic acid. Fed Proc 1958; 17:1075–1077

Miller D, O'Connor P, Williams J. Use of Na-hyaluronate during intraocular lens implantation in rabbits. Ophthalmic Surg 1977; 8:58–61

Miller D, Stegmann R. Use of Na-hyaluronate in corneal transplantation. J Ocular Ther and Surg 1981; 1:28

Miller DM, Stegmann R (eds). Treatment of Anterior Segment Ocular Trauma. Montreal, Medicopea, 1982

Miyake K, Ota I, Ichihashi S, Miyake S, Tanaka T, Terasaki, H. New classification of capsular block syndrome. J Cataract Refract Surg 1998; 24:1230-1234

Miyauchi S, Iwata S. Biochemical studies on the use of sodium hyaluronate in the anterior eye segment. IV. The protective efficacy on the corneal endothelium. Curr Eye Res 1984; 3:1063–1067

Miyauchi S, Iwata S. Evaluations on the usefulness of viscous agents in anterior segment surgery. I. The ability to maintain the deepness of the anterior chamber. J Ocular Pharm 1986; 2:267–274

Miyauchi S, Iwata S. Biochemical studies on the use of sodium hyaluronate in the anterior eye segment. II. The molecular behavior of sodium hyaluronate injected into anterior chamber of rabbits. Curr Eye Res 1987; 3:611–617

Monson MC, Tamura M, Momalis N, Olson RJ. Protective effects of Healon and Occucoat against air bubble endothelial damage during ultrasonic agitation of the anterior chamber. J Cataract Refract Surg 1991; 17:613–616

Mori S. Experimental study on the substitute of the vitreous body. Part 4: Clinical use of some substitutes of the vitreous body. Acta Soc Ophthalmol Jap 1967; 71:22–26

Mortimer C, Sutton H, Henderson C. Efficacy of polyacrylamide vs. sodium hyaluronate in cataract surgery. Can J Ophthalmol 1991; 26:144–147

Müller-Jensen K. Polyacrylamid as an alloplastic vitreous implant. Greafe's Arch Clin Ophthalmol 1974; 189:147–158

Næser K, Thim K, Hansen TE, Degn T, Madsen S, Skov J. Intraocular pressure in the first days after implantation of posterior chamber lenses with the use of sodium hyaluronate (Healon®). Acta Ophthalmol (Copenh) 1986; 64:330–337

Nelson JD, Farris RL. Sodium hyaluronate and polyvinyl alcohol artificial tear preparations: A comparison in patients with keratoconjuncitvitis sicca. Arch Ophthalmol 1988; 106:484–487

Neuhann Th. Capsulorhexis. In: Steinert R. (ed): Cataract Surgery: technique, complications S. 134–142

Nevyas AS, Raber IM, Eagle RC Jr, Wallace IB, Nevyas HJ. Acute band keratopathy following intracameral Viscoat. Arch Ophthalmol 1987; 105:958–964

Nguyen LK, Yee RW, Sigler SC, Ye H-S. Use of in vitro models of bovine corneal endothelial cells to determine the relative toxicity of viscoelastic agents. J Cataract Refract Surg 1992; 18:7–13

Nimrod A, Ezra E, Ezov N, Nachum G, Parisada B. Absorption, distribution, metabolism, and excretion of bacteria-derived hyaluronic acid in rats and rabbits. J Ocular Pharmacol 1992; 8:161–172

Norn MS. Peroperative protection of cornea and conjunctiva. Acta Ophthalmol (Copenh) 1981; 59:587–594

Nuyts RM, Edelhauser HF, Pels E, Breebaart AC. Toxic effects of detergents on the corneal endothelium. Arch Ophthalmol 1990; 108:1158–1162

Özmen A, Guthoff R, Winter R, Draeger J. Vergleichende Untersuchungen zum Einsatz von viskoelastischen Substanzen in der Kataraktchirurgie. Klin Monatsbl Augenheilkd 1992; 200:171–174

Øhrstrm A, Mortensen J, Snne H, Winkler A, Relesj A, Kristoffersen M. A comparison between Amvisc and Healon. Acta Ophthalmol (Copenh) 1993; 71:567–568

Olivius E, Thornburn W. Intraocular pressure after cataract surgery with Healon. J Am Intraocul Implant Soc 1985; 11:480–482

Olson RJ. Cartridge cracks with different viscoelastic agents (letter). J Cataract Refract Surg 1999; 25:465–466

Oosterhuis JA, van Haeringen NJ, Jeltes IG, Glasius E. Polygeline as a vitreous substitute. I. observations in rabbits. Arch Ophthalmol 1966; 76:258–265

Osher Robert H, Cionni RJ, Cohen JS. Re-forming the flat anterior chamber with Healon®. J Cataract Refract Surg 1996; 22:411–415

Packer AJ, Folk JC, Weingeist TA, Goldsmith JC. Procoagulant effects of intraocular sodium hyaluronate. Am J Ophthalmol 1985;100:479–480

Pandolfi M, Hedner U. The effect of sodium hyaluronate and sodium chondroitin sulfate on the coagulation system in vitro. Ophthalmology 1984; 91:864–866

Pape LG. Intracapsular and extracapsular technique of lens implantation with Healon®. J Am Intraocul Implant Soc 1980a; 6:342–343

Pape LG, Balazs EA. The uses of sodium hyaluronate (Healon®) in human anterior segment surgery. Ophthalmology 1980b; 87:699–705

Passo MS, Ernst JT, Goldstick TK. Hyaluronate increases intraocular pressure when used in cataract extraction. Br J Ophthalmol 1985; 69:572–575

Pedersen O. Comparison of the protective effects of methylcellulose and sodium hyaluronate on corneal swelling following phacoemulsification of senile cataracts. J Cataract Refract Surg 1990; 16:594–596

Percival SPB. Complications from use of sodium hyaluronate (Healonid) in anterior segment surgery. Br J Ophthalmol 1982; 66:714–716

Pfeiffer N. Rückblick zur Glaukomforschung. Klin Montasbl Augenheilkd 1993; 203:1–9

Polack FM, Demong T, Santaella H. Sodium hyaluronate (Healon®) in keratoplasty and IOL implantation. Ophthalmology 1981; 88:425–431

Polack FM. Penetrating keratoplasty using MK-stored corneas and Na-hyaluronate (Healon®). Cornea 1982; 1:105–113

Polack FM, McNiece MT. Treatment of dry eyes with Na hyaluronate (Healon®): a preliminary report. Cornea 1982; 1:133–136

Polack FM. Healon (Na hyaluronate): A review of the literature. Cornea 1986; 5:81–93

Poole TA, Sudarsky RD. Suprachoroidal implantation for the treatment of retinal detachment. Ophthalmology 1986; 93:1408–1412

Poyer JF, Chan KY, Arshinoff SA. New method to measure the retention of viscoelastic agents on a rabbit corneal endothelial cell line after irrigation and aspiration. J Cataract Refract Surg 1998; 24:84–90

Poyer JF, Chan KY, Arshinoff SA. Quantitative method to determine the cohesion of viscoelastic agents by dynamic asperation. J Cataract Refract Surg 1998; 24:1130-1135

Prehm P. Hyaluronate is synthesized at plasma membranes. Biochem J 1984; 220:597–600

Probst LE, Nichols BD. Corneal endothelial and intraocular pressure changes after phacoemulsification with Amvisc Plus and Viscoat. J Cataract Refract Surg 1993; 19:725–730

Probst LE, Hakim OJ, Nichols BD. Phacoemulsification with aspirated or retained Viscoat®. J Cataract Refract Surg 1994; 20:145–149

Pruett RC, Calabria GA, Schepens CL. Collagen vitreous substitute. I. Experimental Study. Arch Ophthalmol 1972; 88:540–543

Rafuse PE, Nichols BD. Effects of Healon® vs. Viscoat® on endothelial cell count and morphology after phacoemulsification and posterior chamber lens implantation. Can J Ophthalmol 1992; 27:125–129

Raitta C, Setälä K. Trabeculectomy with the use of sodium hyaluronate: a prospective study. Acta Ophthalmol (Copenh) 1986; 64:407–413

Raitta C, Lehto I, Puska P, Vesti E, Harju M. A randomized, prospective study on the use of sodium hyaluronate (Healon®) in trabeculectomy. Ophthalmic Surg 1994; 25:536–539

Rashid ER, Waring GO III. Use of Healon® in anterior segment trauma. Ophthalmic Surg 1982; 13:201–203

Rath R, Singh AD, Singh A. Cartridge cracks during foldable intraocular lens insertion (letter). J Cataract Refract Surg 1999; 25:306

Ravalico G, Tognetto, Baccara F, Lovisato A. Corneal endothelial protection by different viscoelastics during phacoemulsification. J Cataract Refract Surg 1997; 23:433–439

Raymond L, Jacobson B. Isolation and inhibitory cell growth factors in bovine vitrous. Exp Eye Res 1982; 34:267–286

Reed DB, Mannis MJ, Hills JF, Johnson CA. Corneal epithelial healing after penetrating keratoplasty using topical Healon® versus balanced salt solution. Opthalmic Surg 1987; 18:525–528

Reim M, Saric D. Treatment of chemical burns of the anterior segment with macromolecular sodium hyaluronate (Healon). Rosen ES (ed): Viscoelastic Materials: Basic Science and Clinical Applications. New York, Pergamon Press, 1989, S. 203–215

Roberts B, Pfeiffer RL Jr. Experimental evaluation of a synthetic viscoelastic material on intraocular pressure and corneal endothelium. J Cataract Refract Surg 1989; 15:321–326

Rodriquez F. Principles of polymer systems. New York: Hemisphere Publishing Corporation, 1982:326

Röver J. Phakoemulsifikation des abgesunkenen Linsenkernes im Glaskörperraum. Klin Monatsbl Augenheilkd 1995; 206:456–459

Roper-Hall MJ. Visco elastic materials in the surgery of ocular trauma. Trans Ophthalmol Soc UK 1983; 103:274–276

Rosen ES, Gregory RPF, Barnett F. Is 2% hydroxypropylmethylcellulose a safe solution for intraoperative clinical applications? J Cataract Refract Surg 1986; 12:679–684

Rosen ES, Gregory RPF. Some observations on hydroxypropyl methylcellulose. Rosen ES (ed): Viscoelastic Materials: Basic Science and Clinical Applications. New York, Pergamon Press, 1989, S. 31–37

Roy M, Chen JC, Miller M, Boyaner D, Kasner O, Edelstein E. Epidemic bacillus endophthalmitis after cataract surgery – acute presentation and outcome. Ophthalmology 1997; 104:1768–1772

Salvo EC, Luntz MH, Medow MB. Use of viscoelastic post-trabeculedomy: a survey of members of the American Glancoma Society. Ophthalmic Surg Lasers 1999; 30:271-275

Sand BB, Marner K, Norn MS. Sodium hyaluronate in the treatment of keratoconjunctivitis sicca. Acta Ophthal 1989; 67:181–183

Savage JA, Thomas JV, Belcher CD III, Simmons RJ. Extracapsular cataract extraction and posterior chamber intraocular lens implantation in glaucomatous eyes. Ophthalmology 1985; 92:1506–1516

Scheie HG. Filtration operations for glaucoma: A comparative study. Am J Ophthalmol 1962: 53:571–590

Schmidl B, Mester U, Anterist A. Intraindivdueller Vergleich zweier Viskoelastika unterschiedlicher Viskosität und Molekülgröße (Healon GV, Provisc) bezüglich des Hornhautendothelschutzes bei Phacoemulsifikation an Risikoaugen mit cornea guttata. Ophthalmologe 1998; 95(Suppl):48

Schubert H, Denlinger JL, Balazs EA. Exogenous Na-hyaluronate in the anterior chamber of the owl monkey and its effect on intraocular pressure. Exp Eye Res 1984; 39:137–152

Schwenn O, Müller H, Pfeiffer N, Grehn F. Effects of postfiltration ocular hypotony on visual acuity. Invest Ophthalmol Vis Sci 1997; 38/4:1066

Schwenn O, Pfeiffer N. Keratoplastik und Glaukom. Sitzungsbericht der 159. Versammlung des Vereins Rheinisch-Westfälischer Augenärzte 1997; 77–81

Schwenn O, Dick B, Pfeiffer N. Trabekulotomie, tiefe Sklerektomie und Viskokanalostomie. Nicht fistulierende mikrochirurgische Glaukomoperationen ab externo. Ophthalmologe 1988; 95:835-843

Schwenn O, Dick HB, Krummenauer F, Christmann S, Vogel A, Pfeiffer N. Healon®5 versus Viscoat® during cataract surgery: intraocular pressure, laser flare and corneal changes. Graefe's Arch Clin Exp Ophthalmol 2000; (accepted)

Scott J. The use of visco elastic materials in the posterior segment. Trans Ophthalmol Soc UK 1983; 103:208-283

Scuderi G. Ricerche sperimentali sul trapianto del vitreo. Tentativi di sostituzione parziale con vitreo omologo con liquor eterologo, con soluzioni di polivinil pirrolidone. Ann Ophthal 1954; 80:213

Searl SS, Metz HS, Lindahl KJ. The use of sodium hyaluronate on a biologic sleeve in strabismus surgery. Ann Ophthalmol 1987; 19:259-262

Severin M, Hartmann C. Die Anwendung von Natriumhyaluronat 1% (Healon®) bei der perforierenden Keratoplastik. In: Meyer-Schwickerath G (Hrsg). Viskochirurgie des Auges. Stuttgart, Enke, 1984

Sharp J. What do we mean by „sterility"? J Pharm Sci Technol 1995; 49:90–92

Sharpe ED, Simmons RJ. A prospective comparison of AmviscTM and Healon® in cataract surgery. J Cataract Refract Surg 1986; 12:47–49

Shaw M. Interpretation of osmotic pressure in solutions of one and two nondiffusable components. Biophys J 1976; 16:43–57

Sholiton DB, Solomon OD. Surgical management of black ball hyphema with sodium hyaluronate. Ophthalmic Surg 1981; 12:820–822

Siegel MJ, Spiro HJ, Miller JA, Siegel LI. Secondary glaucoma and uveitis associated with Orcolon (letter). Arch Ophthalmol 1991; 109:1496–1497

Silver FH, Brizzi J, Pins G, Wang M-C, Benedetto D. Physical properties of hyaluronic acid and hydroxypropylmethylcellulose in solution: evaluation of coating ability. J Appl Biomat 1994; 5:89–98

Singh AD, Fang T, Rath R. Cartridge cracks during foldable intraocular lens insertion. J Cataract Refract Surg 1998; 24:1220-1222

Smith KD, Burt WL. Fluorescent viscoelastic enhancement. J Cataract Refract Surg 1992; 18:572–576

Smith SG, Lindstrom RL, Miller RA, Hazel S, Skelnik D, Williams P, Mindrup E. Safety and efficacy of 2% methylcellulose in cat and monkey cataract-implant surgery. J Am Intraocular Implant Soc 1984; 10:160–163

Smith SG, Lindstrom RL. 2% hydroxypropyl methylcellulose as a viscous surgical adjunct – a multicenter prospective randomized trial. J Cataract Refract Surg 1991; 17:839–842

Soll DB, Harrison SE, Arturi FC, Clinch T. Evaluation and protection of corneal endothelium. J Am Intraocul Implant Soc 1980; 6:239–242

Soll DB, Harrison SE. The use of chondroitin sulfate in protection of the corneal endothelium. Ophthalmology 1981; 88(Suppl.):51

Speicher L, Göttinger W. Optische Eigenschaften viskoelastischer Substanzen. Spektrum Augenheilkd 1998; 12:68–69

Stamper RL, DiLoreto D, Schacknow P. Effect of intraocular aspiration of sodium hyaluronate on postoperative intraocular pressure. Ophthalmic Surg 1990; 21:486–491

Steele ADM. Viscoelastic materials in keratoplasty. Trans Ophthalmol Soc UK 1983; 103: 268–269

Steele EA. Hydroxypropyl methylcellulose used as a viscoelastic fluid in ocular surgery, in Rosen ES (ed): Viscoelastic Materials: Basic Science and Clinical Applications. New York, Pergamon Press, 1989, S. 161–163

Stegmann R, Miller D. Protective function of sodium hyaluronate in corneal transplantation. J Ocular Ther Surg 1981; 1:28–31

Stegmann R, Miller D. Extracapsular cataract extraction with sodium hyaluronate. Ann Ophthalmol 1982; 14:813–815

Stegmann R, Miller D. Use of sodium hyaluronate in severe penetrating ocular trauma. Ann Ophthalmol 1986; 18:9–13

Stegmann R, Pienaar A, Miller D. Visco cunalo stormy for open-angle glaucoma in black African patients. J Cataract Refract Surg 1999; 25:316-322

Stenevi U, Gwin T, Härfstrand A, Apple D. Demonstration of hyaluronic acid binding to corneal endothelial cells in human eye-bank eyes. Eur J Implant Refract Surg 1993; 5:228–232

Stenkula S, Ivert L, Gislason I, Tornquist R, Weijdegard L. The use of sodiumhyaluronate (Healon®) in the treatment of retinal detachment. Ophthalmic Surg 1981; 12:435–437

Stenkula S. Sodium hyaluronate as a vitreous substitute and intravitreal surgical tool. Rosen ES (ed): Viscoelastic Materials: Basis Science and Clinical Applications. New York, Pergamon Press, 1989, S. 157–160

Stenzel KH, Dunn MW, Rubin AL. Collagen gels; design for vitreous replacement. Science 1969; 164:1282

Steuhl KP, Weidle EG, Rohrbach JM. Zur operativen Behandlung der hyperplastisch persistierenden Pupillarmembran. Klin Monatsbl Augenheilkd 1992; 201:38–41

Strobel J. Comparison of space-maintaining capabilities of Healon and Healon GV during phacoemulsification. J Cataract Refract Surg 1997; 23:1081–1084

Swartz M, Anderson DR. Use of Healon in posterior segment surgery. J Ocul Ther Surg 1984; 3:26–28

Tan AK, Humphry RC. The fixed dilated pupil after cataract surgery – is it related to intraocular use of hypromellose? Br J Ophthalmol 1993; 77:639–641

Tetz MR, Holzer MP. Two-compartment technique to remove Ophthalmic viscosurgical devices. J Cataract Refr Surg 2000; 26 (accepted for publication)

Thomsen M, Simonsen AH, Andreassen TT. Comparison of sodium hyaluronate and methylcellulose in extracapsular cataract extraction. Acta Ophthalmol (Copenh) 1987; 65:400–405

Toczolowski JR. The use of sodium hyaluronate (Hyalcon) for the removal of severely subluxated lenses. Ophthalmic Surg 1987; 18:214–216

Tofukuji S. Biochemical effects of viscoelastic materials on the glycosaminoglycans in the organ-cultured rabbit trabecular meshwork. Ophthalmologica 1994; 208:1–4

Ullmann S, Lichtenstein SB, Heerlein K. Corneal opacities secondary to Viscoat®. J Cataract Refract Surg 1986; 12:489–492

Van Brunt J. More to hyaluronic acid than meets the eye. Biotechnology 1986; 4:780–782

Vatne HO, Syrdalen P. The use of sodium hyaluronate (Healon®) in the treatment of complicated cases of retinal detachment. Acta Ophthalmol 1986; 64:169–172

Verstraeten TC, Wilcox DK, Friberg TR, Reel C. Effects of silicone oil and hyaluronic acid on cultured human retinal pigment epthelium. Invest Ophthalmol Vis Sci 1990; 31:1761–1766

Völker-Dieben HJ, Regensburg H, Kruit PJ. A double-blind, randomized study of Healon®GV compared with Healon in penetrating keratoplasty. Cornea 1994; 13:414–417

Vörösmarthy D. Okulopressor, ein Instrument zur Erzeugung intraokularer Hypotonie. Klin Monatsbl Augenheilkd 1967; 151:376–382

Wand M. Viscoelastic agent and the prevention of post-filtration flat anterior chamber. Ophthal Surg 1988; 19:523–524

Watson PG. Trabeculectomy, a modified ab externo technique. Ann Ophthalmol 1970; 2:199–205

Watson PG, Barnett F. Effectiveness of trabeculectomy in glaucoma. Am J Ophthalmol 1975; 79:831–845

Wedrich A, Menapace R. Intraocular pressure following small-incision cataract surgery and polyHEMA posterior chamber lens implantation. A comparison between acetylcholine and carbachol. J Cataract Refract Surg 1992; 18:500–505

Wenzel M, Rochels R. Zum derzeitigen Stand der Katarakt- und refraktiven Hornhautchirurgie – Ergebnisse der Umfrage der DGII 1994. In: 9. Kongreß der Deutschsprachigen Gesellschaft für Intraokularlinsen-Implantation und refraktive Chirurgie; (Hrsg: Rochels R, Duncker G, Hartmann Ch). Berlin, Heidelberg, New York, Springer, 1996; S. 3–8

Wenzel M, Ohrloff C, Duncker G. Zum derzeitigen Stand der Katarakt- und refraktiven Hornhautchirurgie – Ergebnisse der Umfrage der DGII 1994. In: 11. Kongreß der Deutschsprachigen Gesellschaft für Intraokularlinsen-Implantation und refraktive Chirurgie; (Hrsg: Ohrloff C, Kohnen T, Duncker G). Berlin, Heidelberg, New York, Springer, 1998; S. 15–20

Weidle EG, Lisch W, Thiel H-J. Management of the opacified posterior lens capsule: an excision technique for membranous changes. Ophthalmic Surg 1986; 17:635–640

Wesendahl TA, Auffarth GU, Sakabe I, Apple DJ. Entfernung viskoelastischer Substanzen nach Linsenimplantation: Eine experimentelle Studie an menschlichen Autopsieaugen. In: Pham DT, Wollensak J, Rochels R, Hartmann Ch. (Hrsg). 8. Kongreß der Deutschsprachigen Gesellschaft für Intraokularlinsen Implantation. Berlin Heidelberg New York, Springer, 1994:446–452

Wilson RP, Lloyd J. The place of sodium hyaluronate in glaucoma surgery. Ophthalmic Surg 1986; 17:30–33

Winter R. Indications for Healon® and installation in microsurgery of complicated retinal detachments. Dev Ophthalmol 1987; 14:20–24

Wirt H, Bill A, Draeger J. Neue Aspekte in der operativen Behandlung des Glaukoms. Vergleich viskoelastischer Substanzen in der Kammerwinkelchirurgie. Ophthalmologe 1992; 89:218–222

Zaidi AA. Trabeculectomy: a review and 4-year follow up. Br J Ophthalmol 1980; 64:436–439

Index

chemical
- composition 18
- properties 16
Chiron Endocoat™ 17
chondroitin sulfate 2, 14, 17–19, 21, 26, 30
choroideal hemorrhage 85
chromatography 31
clarity 7
coatability 7, 8, 15, 53, 55
Coatel 35, 40, 41, 43, 46, 48, 114
coating 14, 76
- ability 15, 30, 39, 53
- capacity 19, 29
- medium 86
cohesive dispersion index (CDI) 15
cohesiveness 15
Collagel 31
collagen 2, 20, 31, 83
- pork collagen 31
colloid osmotic pressure 16, 17, 18
company information 16
compartments, two compartments technique
96
complex
- modulus 35
- viscosity 36
complications 21, 61–64
compression 54
concentration 8, 10–12, 14, 16, 17, 20, 29, 34
conformation 14
congenital glaucoma 82
contact
- angle 7, 15, 53, 86
- gel 86
contamination 21
contractile elements 61
cornea guttata 45, 54
corneal
- dehydration 21
- edema 18
- endothelial protection 53
- epithelium 14, 18
  - epithelial damage 14
- swelling 47
- thickness 18, 47, 57
- transplantation 56
crystalline
- complexes 29
- deposits 22
cyclodialysis 82

D
deformation 8, 9, 11
dehydration / dehydrating effects 18, 56
dermatan sulfate 26
Descemet's membrane 82, 83
dextransulfate 2
dextrose 19
diffraction 66, 72

disaccharide 19
- sub-units 18
Dispasan 16, 21, 22, 34, 40, 41, 43, 46, 48, 108, 120, 121
Dispasan Plus 34, 40, 41, 43, 46, 48, 55, 108, 121
dispersive 3, 4, 15, 59, 72, 73, 74, 94, 95, 96
dissection 70, 82
dissolution 98
distance 10, 50
drag force 54
drug 101, 102
drying 98
dynamic viscosity 8
dystrophy, corneal 58

E
ECCE (extra capsular cataract extraction) 38
elasticity 11, 12, 15, 50, 54
- modulus 35, 36, 45
electrolyte content 16
Ellis-fit 36
endophthalmitis 22
endothelium IV, XVI, 2, 7, 13, 14, 18, 25, 26, 27, 28, 30, 31, 46, 50, 52, 53, 54, 55, 56, 57, 58, 65, 66, 69, 70, 72, 74, 80, 82, 83, 89, 90, 94, 96, 101, 103
endotoxin 21, 23, 29
- concentration 97
enzymatic digestion 29
EU-Working Commission 101
excitation 44
exotoxin 29
extracellular matrix 30
eye drops 87
eye muscles 86

F
FDA 29
fermentation, biological 97
fibrinogen 20
filling 98, 99
filter 24, 99
flexibility 20
flow 10
- behaviour 12
- characteristics 8
- resistance 8
fluid density 10
foldable lenses 39
- intraocular (IOLs) 45, 76
folding forceps 76, 77
force 8, 54, 55
- drag 54
- shear 8, 54, 55
- tractive 55
free radicals 53
frequency 11, 12
Fuchs endothelial dystrophy 45